A–Z of Emergency Radiology

To my mother Darshan. She was a constant source of support, humour and strength through my turmoil-ridden childhood. Without her I would not be where I am today, and I most certainly would not have accomplished what I have.

R.R.M.

To my mother Sally. Without her I would not be the person that I am. Her drive and work ethic are much to be admired, and have had a positive lasting influence upon me.

E.J.H.

A–Z of Emergency Radiology

by
Erskine J. Holmes, MRCS
Specialist Registrar in Accident & Emergency Medicine
Oxford Rotational Training Programme

Rakesh R. Misra, BSc (Hons), FRCS, FRCR
Consultant Radiologist
Wycombe Hospital
Buckinghamshire

A–Z Series Editor
Rakesh R. Misra

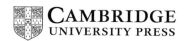
CAMBRIDGE
UNIVERSITY PRESS

CAMBRIDGE UNIVERSITY PRESS

Cambridge, New York, Melbourne, Madrid, Cape Town, Singapore, São Paulo

Cambridge University Press
The Edinburgh Building, Cambridge CB2 2RU, UK

Published in the United States of America by Cambridge University Press, New York

www.cambridge.org
Information on this title: www.cambridge.org/9780521691529

First published 2004
Reprinted by Cambridge University Press 2006

Printed in the United Kingdom at the University Press, Cambridge

A catalogue record for this publication is available from the British Library

ISBN-13 978-0-521-69152-9 paperback
ISBN-10 0-521-69152-4 paperback

Contents

Contents

Preface

Radiology plays an integral role in various medical specialities, with Accident and Emergency (A&E) being no exception. The nature of A&E medicine is such that a clinician encounters a potentially huge variety of pathologies in any one shift. Consequently, the various radiological investigations requested in the A&E setting often form the cornerstone of accurate patient management.

Many established textbooks are available in Medicine, Surgery and Paediatrics for example, which detail the management of various disease processes. Similarly there are textbooks of radiology that detail the radiology of the same. However, it is not uncommon for a clinician to require both the management and radiology immediately to hand when confronted by a sick patient. This is where we hope this book comes in.

The book is divided into conveniently recognised body sections; *head and face, cervical spine, thorax, abdomen, upper limb* and *lower limb*. Within each section we have covered a 'core' set of diagnoses that regularly present themselves to A&E and, where possible, have subdivided each diagnosis according to *characteristic, clinical features, radiological features* and *management*. The supplied radiographs have been chosen both for their high quality and as excellent examples of the conditions being described.

We have intentionally avoided being over-expansive with the text in this book, as it is intended to be a concise overview to emergency radiology and is meant to help expedite a patient's passage through the A&E setting. It is with this in mind that we feel this work is not only suited to both undergraduate students and doctors at all stages of their training, but also to A&E nurse practitioners and to other ancillary medical staff involved in emergency medicine.

R. R. M.
E. J. H.
April 2004

Acknowledgements

We would like to acknowledge the contribution made by Mr James Murray, MRCS. Many an hour was spent by James reading through the text and his contribution is much appreciated.

List of abbreviations

ABCs	–	Airway, breathing, circulation (according to ATLS protocol)
AC	–	Acromio-clavicular
A&E	–	Accident and emergency
AP	–	Antero-posterior
ASB	–	Anatomical snuff box
ATLS	–	Advanced trauma life support
AXR	–	Abdominal X-ray
BiPAP	–	Bidirectional positive airway pressure
COPD	–	Chronic obstructive pulmonary disease
CSF	–	Cerebrospinal fluid
CT	–	Computed tomography
CXR	–	Chest radiograph
DPL	–	Diagnostic peritoneal lavage
ECG	–	Electrocardiogram
ESR	–	Erythrocyte sedimentation rate
ENT	–	Ear, nose, throat
GA	–	General anaesthesia
GCS	–	Glasgow coma scale
ICH	–	Intracranial haemorrhage
ICP	–	Intracranial pressure
i.v.	–	Intravenous
IVC	–	Inferior vena cava
IVP	–	Intravenous pyelogram
KUB	–	Kidney, ureter, bladder
MRI	–	Magnetic resonance imaging
NAI	–	Non-accidental injury
NG	–	Nasogastric
NOF	–	Neck of femur
NSAIDs	–	Non-steroidal anti-inflammatory drugs
OPG	–	Orthopantomogram
PA	–	Postero-anterior
PC	–	Pelvicalyceal system
PEEP	–	Positive end expiratory pressure
PUO	–	Pyrexia of unknown origin
RLQ	–	Right lower quadrant
SAH	–	Subarachnoid haemorrhage
SDH	–	Subdural haematoma
SMV	–	Submentovertex
SUFE	–	Slipped upper femoral epiphysis

List of abbreviations

TC	–	Transverse colon
TIA	–	Transient ischaemic attack
TMJ	–	Temporomandibular joint
TB	–	Tuberculosis
WCC	–	White cell count
US	–	Ultrasound
#	–	Fracture

Proposed algorithms

Algorithm for the management of head injury in children <2 years

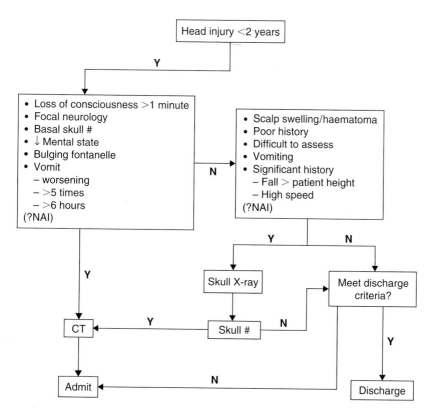

Discharge criteria

1. NO neurological symptoms
2. NO significant extra cranial injuries/illness
3. NO suspicion of neglect/abuse
4. Reliable parents/guardians
5. Appropriate discharge advise
6. No parental concerns re-behaviour
7. Have good access to hospital (transport/location)

NB: If unsure, ask senior advice.

Proposed algorithms

Algorithm for the management of head injury in children <16 years

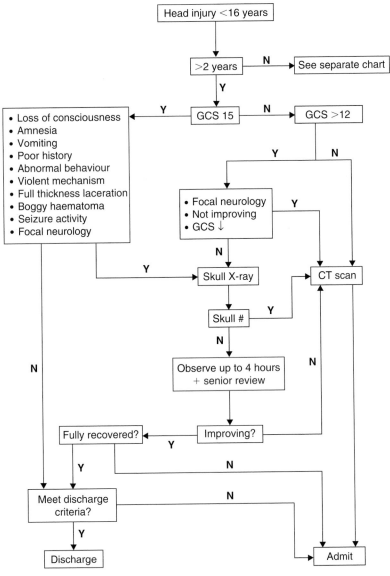

Head injury <16 years

>2 years — N → See separate chart

Y

GCS 15 — N → GCS >12

Y →
- Loss of consciousness
- Amnesia
- Vomiting
- Poor history
- Abnormal behaviour
- Violent mechanism
- Full thickness laceration
- Boggy haematoma
- Seizure activity
- Focal neurology

N

Y

- Focal neurology
- Not improving
- GCS ↓

Y → CT scan

N

Skull X-ray → CT scan

Skull # — Y

N

Observe up to 4 hours + senior review

N

Improving?

Fully recovered? ← Y

N

N

Meet discharge criteria?

N

Y

Discharge

Admit

NB: Refer neurosurgery if: CT +ve
GCS <8

NB: The National Institute of Clinical Excellence (www.NICE.org.uk) had recently released guidelines relating to the management of adult head injury.

HEAD AND FACE

Cerebral contusion

Characteristics

- Commonest form of traumatic intra-axial injury.
- Contusions occur at the inferior and polar surfaces of the frontal and temporal lobes.
- Injury results secondary to contact with bony surfaces during deceleration and is produced by damage to parenchymal blood vessels leading to petechial haemorrhage and oedema.
- Contusions develop in surface grey matter tapering into white matter.
- Injuries may be coup or contra-coup.
- Cerebral contusions are also produced secondary to depressed skull fractures and are associated with other intracranial injuries.

Clinical features

- Usually associated with a brief loss of consciousness. Confusion and obtundation may be prolonged.
- Focal neurological deficit can occur if contusions arise near the sensori-motor cortex.
- Most patients make an uneventful recovery but a proportion develop raised intracranial pressure (ICP), post-traumatic seizures and persisting focal deficits.
- Beware of the elderly patients, alcoholics and patients taking anticoagulants as they are at increased risk of haemorrhage.

Radiological features

- Non-contrast computed tomography (CT) useful in the early post-traumatic period.
- Contusions are seen as multiple focal areas of low or mixed attenuation intermixed with tiny areas of increased density representing petechial haemorrhage.
- True extent becomes apparent over time with progression of cell necrosis and oedema.
- Magnetic resonance imaging (MRI) is the best modality for demonstration of oedema and contusion distribution.

Management

- Secure airway whilst the cervical spine is protected. Supplemental oxygen. Assess and stabilise breathing and circulation.
- If Glasgow coma scale (GCS) < 8 discuss with anaesthetist as a definitive (secured) airway is required.
- Early discussion with radiologist and neurosurgeon.
- Titrate opioid analgesia. Cleanse and close scalp injuries. Discuss with a neurosurgeon regarding intravenous (i.v.) antibiotics, steroid and mannitol use.

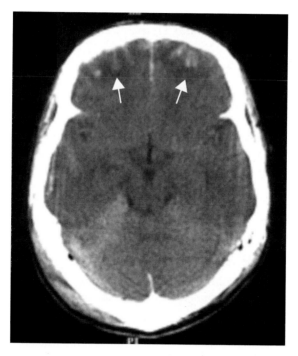

Cerebral contusions in both frontal lobes (arrows). The adjacent low density represents local oedema.

Extradural haematoma

Characteristics

- The majority of these are arterial (middle meningeal artery) with a small proportion being of venous origin.
- Commonly unilateral and associated with a fracture in adults. Skull fractures are often absent in children due to skull elasticity.
- Haematoma forms between the inner table of skull and the dura.
- May have associated injuries, such as a subdural haematoma (SDH) or contusions.
- Arterial bleeding usually develops and presents rapidly within 1 hour of injury whereas venous haematomas may present after several days.

Clinical features

- Classically present following a head injury with initial loss of consciousness followed by a lucid interval, prior to a second decrease in the level of consciousness.
- Beware as only about 30% of patients present in this way.
- The symptomatology depends on how quickly the haematoma expands. Progressive sleepiness, headache, nausea and vomiting are suspicious.

Radiological features

- CT signs include a *biconvex* hyperdense elliptical collection with a sharply defined edge. Mixed density suggests active bleeding.
- The haematoma does not cross suture lines.
- May separate the venous sinuses/falx from the skull; this is the only type of haemorrhage to do this.
- Mass effect depends on the size of the haemorrhage and associated oedema.
- Venous bleeding is more variable in shape.
- Associated fracture line may be seen.

Management

- Airways, breathing, circulation (ABCs).
- Definitive treatment involves surgical evacuation; therefore early discussion with a neurosurgeon is important.

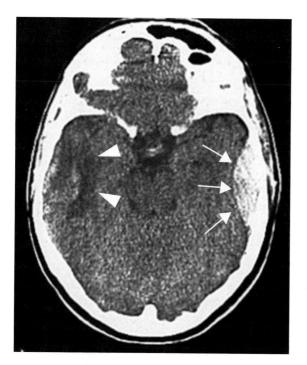

Lentiform-shaped high density left extradural haematoma (arrows). Note the contra-coup right temporal contusions (arrowheads).

Facial fractures

Characteristics

- Often secondary to assault in adults and falls in children. Facial fractures in children are suspicious of non-accidental injury (NAI).
- Emphasis on diagnosis rather than specific treatment in accident and emergency (A&E). Functional loss and disability can be significant following facial trauma.
- Consider cervical spine injury in all.
- Classified according to site – maxillary (sub-classified by Le Fort), malar, infra-orbital, mandibular and nasal.

Clinical features

Maxillary

- Commonly associated with massive facial trauma and other organ trauma. Presents with massive soft tissue swelling, mid-face mobility and malocclusion. Cerebrospinal fluid (CSF) rhinorrhoea may occur secondary to dural tears.
- Significant epistaxis can occur compromising both airway and circulation and can require intervention.

Le Fort classification

Le Fort I	involves tooth bearing maxilla.
Le Fort II	involves maxilla, nasal bones and medial aspects of orbits.
Le Fort III	involves maxilla, nasal bones, vomer, ethmoids and small bones of skull base. **The face is separated from the skull base.**

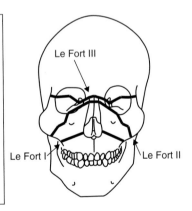

Malar

- The zygoma may fracture in isolation or more commonly extend through to the infra-orbital foramen with disruption of the zygomatico-temporal and zygomatico-frontal sutures (tripod fracture).
- Look for cheek flattening, a palpable step, infra-orbital nerve damage and diplopia.
- Intra-oral examination may reveal bony irregularity above and behind the upper molars.

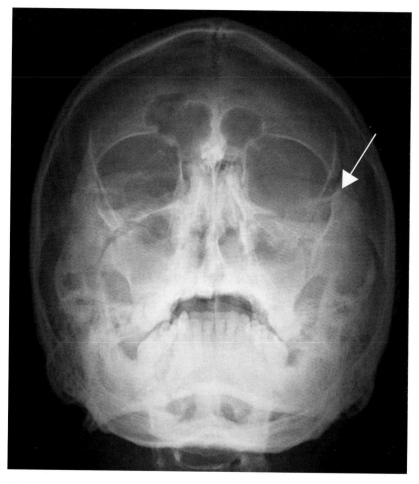

Mid-face fracture – Le Fort II. Additional diastasis of the left zygomatico-frontal suture (arrow).

Facial fractures (continued)

Infra-orbital (blow out) fracture

- Enophthalmos and orbital emphysema may be evident. Diplopia may occur secondary to ocular muscle (or orbital fat) entrapment.
- Globe injuries not uncommon, e.g. retinal detachment.

Mandibular

- Pain and tenderness and a palpable step may be evident. Malocclusion common. May fracture distant to point of impact.
- Lip numbness suggests inferior dental nerve damage.

Radiological features

Maxillary

- Request facial views. Fractures can be difficult to see.
- CT scan often of benefit to delineate number and extent of fractures. Helpful in planning surgery and subsequent follow-up.
- Fractures rarely occur in their pure form and are often asymmetrical.

Malar

- Facial views supplemented by submentovertex (SMV) views to visualise the zygomatic arches.

Infra-orbital

- Facial views may show a 'teardrop', representing soft tissue, herniating into the maxillary sinus. Complete opacification of the maxillary sinus occurs secondary to haemorrhage and oedema and, if unilateral, should be considered to be a secondary fracture until proven otherwise.
- Depression of the orbital floor may be visible.
- Air within the soft tissues may be seen with orbital emphysema.

Mandibular

- Confirm with a panoramic view (orthopantomogram, OPG) with combined antero–posterior (AP) views.
- Condylar views may show a fracture or temporomandibular joint (TMJ) dislocation. Coronal CT is of benefit in difficult to visualise condylar fractures.

Management

General

- ABCs.
- Make the diagnosis from clinical and radiological examination.

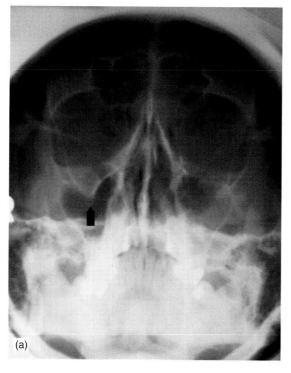

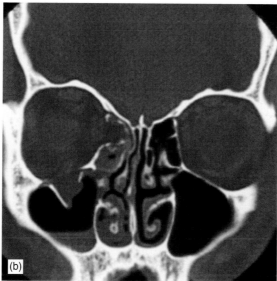

Infra-orbital fracture. (a) 'Teardrop' sign. (b) Coronal CT demonstrating the same.

Facial fractures (*continued*)

- Discuss with ear, nose, throat (ENT) surgeons.
- Antibiotics recommended for open fractures.

Special considerations

- *Maxillary*: Airway compromise is common and requires careful maintenance. Epistaxis may require nasal packing/tampon. Operative intervention for epistaxis is uncommon.
- *Zygomatic*: Depressed zygomatic fractures often require elevation.
- *Infra-orbital*: Spontaneous resolution of signs may occur and thus delayed repair is often performed. In a patient with orbital emphysema with a sudden decrease in visual acuity consider vascular compromise secondary to raised orbital pressure. This is a surgical emergency.
- *Mandibular*: In most cases these require admission for occlusive or mandibular wiring.

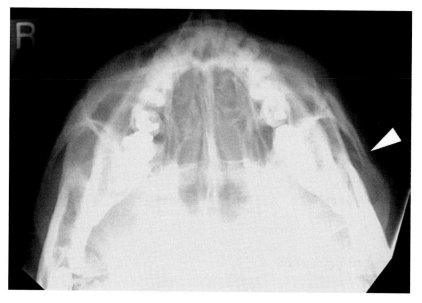

Left zygomatic arch fracture.

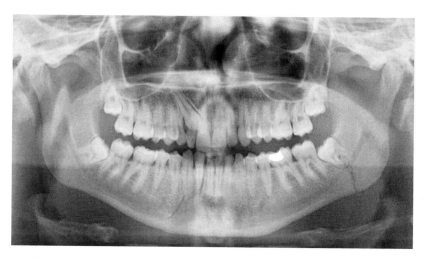

OPG: Fractures of right body and left ramus of mandible.

Skull fracture

Characteristics

- Caused by direct impact to the skull.
- Marker for underlying brain injury as this requires a substantial force.
- Classified as linear, depressed or basal.
- Type depends on amount of force applied and the ratio of force to the impact area.
- Clinically difficult to detect. If detectable there is likely to be underlying brain injury.
- Increased significance if an open fracture, or if the fracture communicates with an air sinus, is depressed or crosses an artery or major dural sinus.
- Beware NAI; commonest cause of skull fracture in an infant.

Clinical features

Linear

- Often no associated underlying brain injury and are thus relatively asymptomatic.
- If fracture line crosses a sinus, a suture or a dural/vascular groove, there is an increased risk of complications such as haemorrhage or infection.

Depressed

- A palpable bony depression may be felt. This can be difficult if an overlying haematoma is present. With an open fracture, the depressed fragment may be missed due to the mobility of the scalp.
- The risk of brain injury increases with the depth of depression. Approximately 25% of patients will present with loss of consciousness. Neurological deficits depend on the underlying brain injury.
- Increased risk of developing seizures and meningitis.

Basal

- Clinical signs include haemotympanum (or blood in the auditory canal), rhinorrhoea, otorrhoea, Battles' sign (retro-auricular haematoma), Racoon eyes (periorbital ecchymosis) and cranial nerve deficits (3rd, 4th and 5th).
- Blotting paper is useful in a patient with a bloody nose to diagnose rhinorrhoea. Placed on blotting paper the CSF will extend further and appear as a lucent ring around the blood.

Radiological features

- Plain skull radiographs are the initial investigation with some progressing to CT.
- *Linear fractures* will appear as a deeply black sharply defined line. May be mistaken for a suture line or vascular groove. A vascular groove often branches, has a sclerotic margin and a typical site.

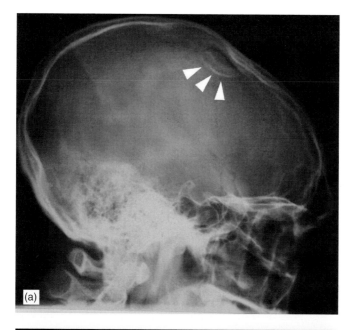

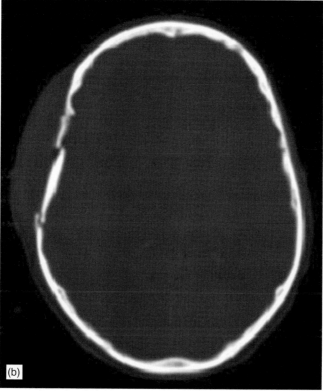

(a) Depressed skull fracture (arrowheads) with (b) CT correlation (different patient).

Skull fracture (*continued*)

- *Depressed fractures* are often difficult to see. Look for increased or double density related either to bony overlap or if the fracture has being imaged tangentially.
- *Basal skull fractures* are not well seen on plain radiographs. Look for fluid level within sphenoid sinus. If suspected the patient should have a CT.
- CT will often demonstrate skull fractures when viewed on bony windows. More useful for visualisation of secondary complications.

Management

- ABCs. Prevent secondary brain injury.
- Admit for observation. The management of the fracture and any subsequent complications should be discussed with a neurosurgeon.
- Most CSF leaks spontaneously resolve within 1 week without complications and thus prophylactic antibiotics should not routinely be given during this time.
- If a fracture segment is depressed below the inner table, elevation is usually required.

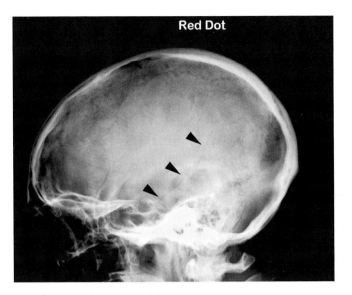

Simple vault fracture (arrowheads).

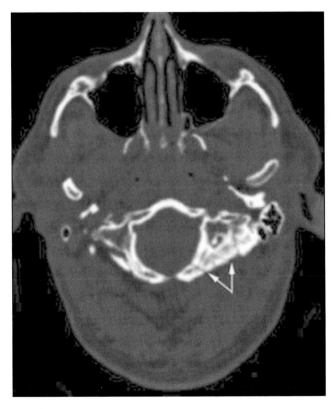

Base of skull fracture (arrows).

Stroke

Characteristics

- Defined as a focal neurological deficit of vascular origin lasting >24 hours. Often preceded by a transient ischaemic attack (TIA) (10–15%).
- Non-specific term encompassing a spectrum of pathophysiological processes.
- May be due to infarction (80%) or haemorrhage (20%).
- Infarction is usually secondary to *in situ* thrombosis, e.g. secondary to atherosclerosis, or embolism (usually of cardiac origin).
- Haemorrhagic strokes are associated with hypertension, usually of long standing duration.
- In both haemorrhagic and ischaemic strokes, local tissue injury leads to oedema and further compromise of blood supply.

Clinical features

- Ischaemic stroke usually presents with a focal neurological deficit. Onset is usually sudden but there may be a step-like progression. Headache, complete loss of consciousness and vomiting are uncommon unless the brain stem is involved.
- Hemisphere injury classically presents with contra-lateral weakness, decreased tone and reflexes, sensory loss and dysphasia.
- Haemorrhagic presentation varies according to site, type and location of the bleed. Headache, vomiting, focal neurological deficit and decreased level of consciousness are characteristic. Beware quick progression to coma.

Radiological features

- Non-contrast CT in the first instance.
- In the first 6 hours an ischaemic stroke is difficult to visualise.
- CT is useful in detecting haemorrhage and also to identify structural lesions mimicking stroke, such as a tumour, subdural/extradural haematomas and abscesses.
- A normal CT *does not* exclude raised ICP.

Management

- ABCs.
- The main management aim is to prevent secondary brain injury. Supportive care is paramount with supplemental oxygen and fluids (avoid over-hydration) as required.
- Think of early airway management for definitive control of the airway and subsequent ventilation and imaging. Traumatic management of the airway will raise ICP.

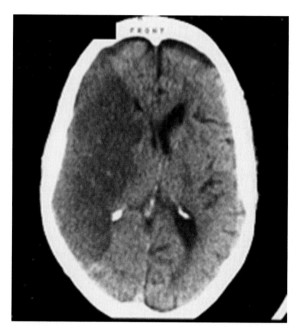

Large area of low density in the right cerebral hemisphere. This represents a right middle cerebral artery territory infarct.

- Optimal blood pressure management in hypertensive patients with suspected intracranial haemorrhage (ICH) is controversial. Be guided by local practice.
- Steroids are not indicated.
- Surgery may be of benefit in cerebellar haemorrhage.
- The use of thrombolysis is not currently recommended.

Subarachnoid haemorrhage

Characteristics

- Spontaneous subarachnoid haemorrhage (SAH) usually occurs secondary to a ruptured aneurysm or arteriovenous malformation.
- Acquired aneurysms are commonest in the circle of Willis; at bifurcations with turbulent flow.
- Commonest before 50 years of age, but may occur at any age.
- Free blood causes irritation of the meninges.
- A sentinel headache occurs in roughly two-third of patients heralding a future bleed.

Clinical features

- Acute severe headache often described as the worst ever, although a mild headache does not exclude a SAH.
- Vomiting, pallor and profuse sweating may occur.
- Neck stiffness and focal neurological signs ± seizures.
- Beware altered level of consciousness that rapidly progresses to coma.
- Complications include hydrocephalus (acute obstructive and delayed communicating), cerebral vasospasm leading to infarction and trans-tentorial herniation secondary to raised ICP.
- Mimics many other conditions including encephalitis, meningitis, acute glaucoma and migraine amongst others.

Radiological features

- Non-contrast CT is sensitive within 4–5 hours of onset.
- Look for acute haemorrhage (increased density) in the cortical sulci, basal cisterns, Sylvian fissures, superior cerebellar cisterns and in the ventricles.
- MRI is relatively insensitive within the first 48 hours but is useful after this time and in recurrent bleeds to pick up subtle haemosiderin deposition.

Management

- ABCs. Beware as patients may rapidly progress to coma and require intubation.
- Supplemental oxygen, i.v. access and cardiac monitoring are essential.
- Consider other causes for a decreased level of consciousness.
- Check routine bloods and refer suspicious patients for further investigation, e.g. lumbar puncture or CT scan.
- A normal CT *does not* exclude a SAH. This group of patients require a lumbar puncture.

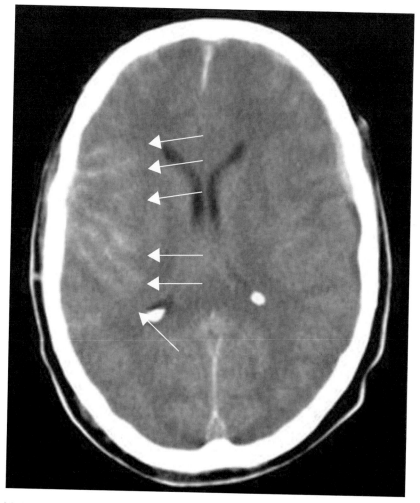

Multiple areas of linear high density are seen within the right cerebral sulci (arrows); these represent areas of acute subarachnoid haemorrhage.

Subdural haematoma

Characteristics

- SDH commonly occurs in the elderly and in children (beware NAI).
- Occur in the subdural space, i.e. the potential space between pia arachnoid membrane and dura.
- Caused by traumatic tearing of bridging veins in the subdural space.
- Often secondary to deceleration injuries, or direct trauma in which there is movement of the brain in relation to the skull. Beware forceful coughing/sneezing or vomiting in the elderly.
- No consistent relationship to skull fractures.

Clinical features

- Often insidious due to the slow build up of pressure. The resultant mass effect over time can lead to significant ischaemic damage.
- Clinical presentation depends on the amount of trauma sustained and the speed of haematoma accumulation.
- Classified as acute or chronic depending on time of presentation.
- Acute SDHs present within 24 hours of injury usually with decreased level of consciousness or a decline in mental status. Signs of mass effect should be looked for.

Radiological features

- CT shows a *crescentic* fluid collection between the brain and inner skull. Concave inner margin with minimal brain substance displacement.
- Crosses suture lines but not dural reflections.
- In the *acute phase* the fluid collections appear to be of high density; in the *subacute phase* (2–4 weeks post-injury) the collection is isodense to brain and in the *chronic phase* (>4 weeks post-injury) the collection is of low density.

Management

- ABCs.
- Discuss with neurosurgeon. Even small haematomas may be suitable for evacuation.
- Conservative management in patients with haematomas only a few millimetres thick may be appropriate after considered discussion and further careful observation.

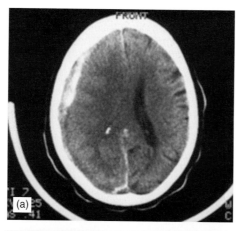

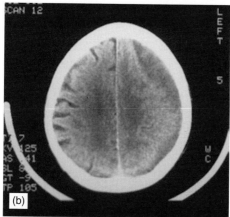

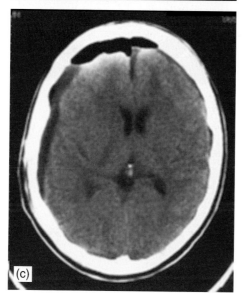

(a) Acute SDH; (b) Subacute SDH; (c) Chronic SDH.

CERVICAL SPINE

Cervical spine injuries

Characteristics

- Majority are seen secondary to road traffic accidents. Falls from heights and sporting accidents make up the second largest category.
- Most commonly seen in young men. A relative increase in incidence is seen in the elderly as arthritis and degenerative changes increase susceptibility.
- Classified according to mechanism of trauma:
  - Flexion injuries
  - Rotational injuries
  - Extension injuries
  - Vertical compression injuries

Flexion injuries

- *Simple wedge fracture*: Compression fracture of the *antero-superior* aspect of the vertebral body. Generally stable unless associated with posterior ligamentous disruption.
- *Teardrop fracture*: Fracture through the *antero-inferior* aspect of the vertebral body, often with anterior displacement of the fragment. Commonly associated with ligamentous disruption and hence the fracture is *unstable*. This differs from an extension teardrop fracture in that the anterior height of the vertebral body is usually reduced, in keeping with the mechanism of injury.
- *Clay shovelers' fracture*: Spinous process fracture following direct trauma or ligamentous avulsion – *stable injury*.
- *Atlanto-occipital and alanto-axial dislocation*: Highly unstable. May be associated with an odontoid fracture.
- *Bilateral facet dislocation*: Requires a large degree of force and is highly unstable. Best seen on the lateral view. The vertebral body above displaces anteriorly by at least 50% of the AP diameter of the vertebral body. The facets often appear 'locked'.
- *Odontoid fracture*: Subdivided according to site. *Type 1* occurs at the tip and is stable. *Type 2* involves the junction of odontoid and vertebral body. *Type 3* occurs through the superior aspect of C2 at the base of the odontoid. Types 2 and 3 are unstable especially if associated with anterior or lateral displacement.
- *Uncinate process fracture*: Occurs secondary to lateral flexion. Stable injury.

Rotational injuries

- *Unilateral facet dislocation*: Usually secondary to a flexion/rotation injury. Superior facet dislocates anteriorly over the inferior facet. Considered a stable injury unless it occurs at the C1/C2 level.

Extension injuries

- *Fracture of posterior arch of the atlas*: Occurs secondary to compressive force between axis and occiput.

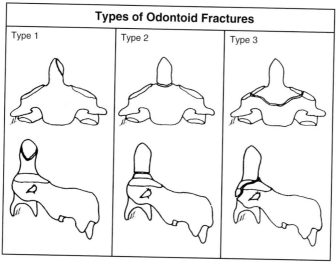

Types of Odontoid Fractures

| Type 1 | Type 2 | Type 3 |

Classification of odontoid peg fractures. From: *Sports Medicines: Problems and Practical Management* (Eds E. Sherry & D. Bokor); Greenwich Medical Media, 1997: page 117.

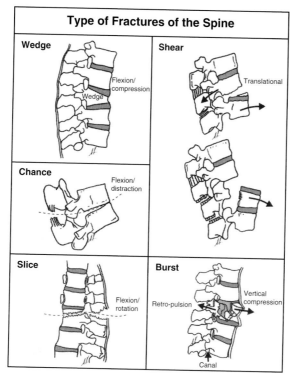

Type of Fractures of the Spine

Wedge — Flexion/compression, Wedge

Shear — Translational

Chance — Flexion/distraction

Slice — Flexion/rotation

Burst — Retro-pulsion, Vertical compression, Canal

Types of fracture of the spine. From: *Sports Medicines: Problems and Practical Management* (Eds E. Sherry & D. Bokor); Greenwich Medical Media, 1997: page 120.

Cervical spine (continued)

- *Teardrop fracture*: The anterior longitudinal ligament avulses the anterio-inferior corner of the vertebral body. Common at C2 and C5–C7. Vertebral body height preserved. This injury is *unstable in extension*.
- *Hangman's fracture*: Bilateral fracture through the pedicles of C2. A degree of subluxation of C2 on C3 occurs. Common in road traffic accidents – an *unstable injury*.

Vertical compression injuries

- *Jefferson fracture*: Occipital condyles force lateral masses of C1 laterally leading to fractures of the anterior and posterior arches with associated transverse ligament rupture – an *unstable injury*.
- *Burst fracture*: Intervertebral disc is driven into the vertebral body below. Fracture fragments may impinge on the cord and thus should be thought of as unstable even though the fracture itself is stable.

Clinical examination

- *All patients with documented, or suspected, trauma above the level of the clavicles should be considered to have a cervical spine injury until proven otherwise.* These patients should have cervical spine immobilisation until cleared both radiologically and clinically.
- Obtain an accurate history if possible prior to examination. The mechanism of injury will often reveal the suspected bony abnormality.
- Examine from 'top to toe' in a systematic way looking for signs of trauma. Speak to the patient, both to reassure and to localise a potential injury, e.g. painful hands can represent an unstable injury at C6/C7!
- The cervical spine can be examined whilst immobilised. Palpate the neck for muscle spasm, mid-line bony tenderness, palpable steps and crepitus.
- Assess the neurological system carefully and document the time and findings.
- A *complete* spinal cord lesion is defined as 'complete loss of motor and sensory function below the level of a spinal cord injury'. If symptoms persist >24 hours the chances of recovery are slim. Spinal shock can mimic the symptoms although this usually recovers in <24 hours.
- *Incomplete* lesions can generally be grouped into three syndromes – central cord lesions, Brown–Sequard syndrome and anterior cord lesions.

Radiological evaluation

- A cervical spine injury is unlikely in an alert patient (i.e. not under the influence of alcohol or drugs) without neck pain, bony tenderness, focal neurological defect or a painful distracting injury.

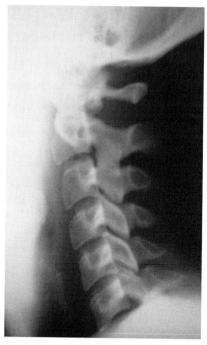 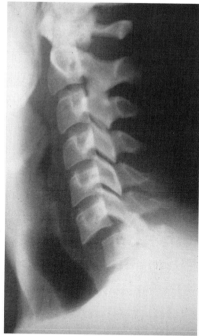

This demonstrates the importance of visualising the whole cervical spine down to the cervico-thoracic junction. Bilateral locked facets at C6/C7.

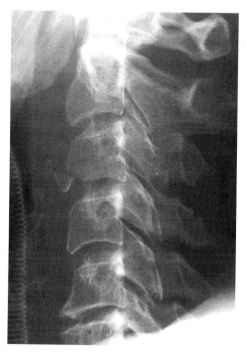

A teardrop fracture at C3.

Cervical spine injuries (continued)

- Obtain lateral, AP and an open mouth peg view if a cervical spine injury is suspected:
  - *Lateral view*: Examine the **ABCS**:
    - **A** *Alignment and adequacy*: Visualise from base of skull to the C7/T1 junction. In-line arm traction, during the cross table lateral or a swimmer's views can be helpful in visualising C7/T1. Look for the normal smooth curve of the anterior vertebral, posterior vertebral and spino–laminar lines (see diagram). In a child pseudo-subluxation of C2 on C3 can cause confusion. In these cases, examine the spino–laminar line from C1 to C3. If the bases of these spinous processes lie >2 mm from this line an injury should be suspected. Correlate with soft tissue findings (see below). The distance between the anterior arch of C1 and the odontoid peg should be <3 mm in an adult and 5 mm in a child.
    - **B** *Bone*: Assess for normal bony outline and density. An increase in density may indicate a compression fracture.
    - **C** *Cartilage*: The intervertebral spaces should be uniform. Widening of these or the interspinous distance may indicate an unstable dislocation. An increase in interspinous distance of >50% suggests ligamentous disruption. Muscular spasm can make interpretation difficult.
    - **S** *Soft tissues*: Retro-pharyngeal soft tissue swelling may be the only sign of a significant injury. Normal measurements are less than 7 mm C2–C4 (half a vertebral body at this level) and less than 22 m below C5 (a vertebral body width). Air within the soft tissues suggests rupture of oesophagus or trachea/bronchus. Bulging of the pre-vertebral fat stripe is an early sign.
  - *AP view*: The tips of the spinous process should lie in a straight line in the mid-line. Bifid spinous processes can make interpretation difficult. Again assess the interspinous distances for ligamentous rupture.
  - *Open mouth view*: The distance between the odontoid and the lateral masses of C1 should be equal. Inequality may be due to head rotation. In such cases the lateral margins should remain aligned. Fractures may be mimicked by congenital anomalies and non-fusion in children. Overlying soft tissues, the occiput and dentition may also mimic a fracture (attempt to trace the suspect line beyond the bony cortical margins).
  - *Other views*: Oblique and flexion/extension views are useful if experienced.
- Remember if a fracture is found there are likely to be other abnormalities!
- CT: Used to further evaluate abnormalities and when plain films are inadequate. Technically superior to plain films in assessing fractures, soft tissues and the spinal canal.
- MRI: Used to assess soft tissues, ligaments and the spinal column.

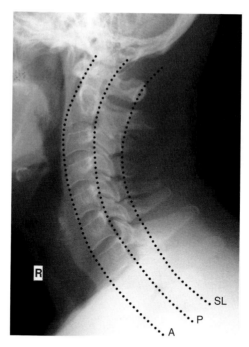

Always assess the anterior vertebral (A), posterior vertebral (P) and spinolaminar (SL) lines.

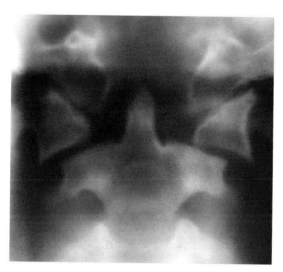

A Jefferson's fracture.

Cervical spine injuries (*continued*)

Management

- ABCs.
- Should the patient need intubating, this can be carried out with in-line immobilisation by one experienced in the technique. Early transfer from a rigid backboard is essential to prevent pressure sores and should be carried out in a co-ordinated manner with the required number of staff.
- With the cervical spine immobilised (the **holy trilogy** of a semi-rigid collar, head blocks and tape) carefully assess for other injuries. Once stabilised, the cervical spine can be assessed with in-line immobilisation. A full documented neurological examination should be carried out. Consult the orthopaedic team early if a cervical spine injury is suspected.
- A normal cross table lateral radiograph does not exclude a spinal cord injury. If in doubt, maintain immobilisation and ask for advice. And *remember*, children have an increased incidence of **S**pinal **C**ord **I**njury **W**ith**o**ut **R**adiographic **A**bnormality (SCIWoRA).

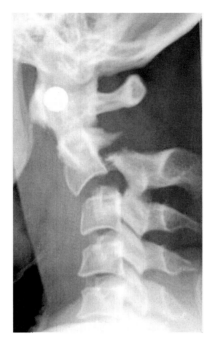

A Hangman's fracture.

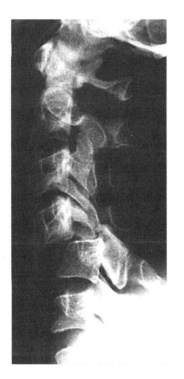

Bilateral locked facets.

THORAX

Aortic rupture

Characteristics

- Eighty to ninety per cent of patients die before reaching hospital.
- Associated with deceleration injuries, such as a fall from a height or in road traffic accidents over 40 mph.
- The aorta usually ruptures at the aortic isthmus (in 88–95%), just distal to the origin of the left subclavian artery.

Clinical features

- An aortic rupture should be suspected from the mechanism of injury.
- Chest or inter-scapular pain will be present.
- Differential brachial blood pressures or different brachial and femoral pulse volumes are suggestive.

Radiological features

Chest radiograph

- Widened mediastinum (>8 cm on a supine AP Chest radiograph (CXR)).
- Blurred aortic outline with loss of aortic knuckle.
- Left apical pleural cap.
- Left sided haemothorax.
- Depressed left/raised right main stem bronchus.
- Tracheal displacement to the right.
- Oesophageal NG tube displacement to the right.

CT Thorax

- Vessel wall disruption or extra-luminal blood seen in contiguity with the aorta is indicative of rupture.

Management

- ABCs.
- Judicious fluid replacement.
- Adequate analgesia.
- Avoid hypertension (excess fluid replacement/pain, etc.).
- Urgent surgical involvement with a view to thoracotomy and repair.

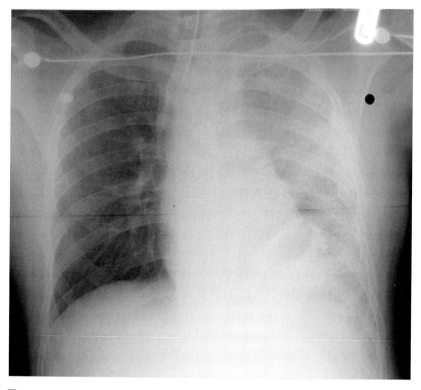

Traumatic aortic rupture: tracheal deviation to the right, depressed left main stem bronchus; left haemothorax, blurring of the outline of the aortic arch and a left pleural apical cap. Rib fractures and a traumatic left diaphragmatic hernia are also noted.

Chronic obstructive pulmonary disease

Characteristics

- General term encompassing a spectrum of conditions including chronic bronchitis and emphysema.
- Characterised by chronic airflow reduction resulting from resistance to expiratory airflow, infection, mucosal oedema, bronchospasm and bronchoconstriction due to reduced lung elasticity.
- Causative factors include smoking, chronic asthma, alpha-1 antitrypsin deficiency and chronic infection.

Clinical features

- Exacerbations commonly precipitated by infection.
- Cough, wheeze and exertional dyspnoea.
- Tachypnoea, wheeze, lip pursing (a form of positive end expiratory pressure, (PEEP)) and use of accessory muscles.
- Cyanosis, plethora and signs of heart failure suggest severe disease.
- Signs of hypercarbia include coarse tremor, bounding pulse, peripheral vasodilatation, drowsiness, confusion or an obtunded patient.

Radiological features

- CXRs are only moderately sensitive (40–60%), but highly specific in appearance.
  - Easily accessible method of assessing the extent and degree of structural parenchymal damage.
  - In the emergency setting, useful for assessing complications, such as pneumonia, heart failure, lobar collapse/atelectasis, pneumothorax or rib fractures.
  - Radiographic features include hyper-expanded lungs with associated flattening of both hemidiaphragms, pruning of pulmonary vasculature, 'barrel-shaped chest' and lung bullae.

Management

- ABCs.
- Supplemental oxygen tailored to keep $pO_2 > 7.5\,kPa$.
- Nebulised bronchodilators (oxygen or air driven where appropriate). Adding nebulised ipratropium bromide may help.
- Consider an aminophylline or salbutamol infusion.
- Corticosteroids unless contraindicated.
- Appropriate antibiotics should be given if infection suspected.
- Ventilation or bidirectional positive airway pressure (BiPAP) should be considered.

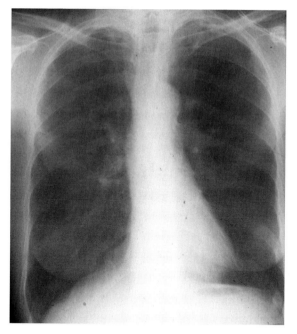

The lungs are hyperinflated with flattening of both hemidiaphragms.

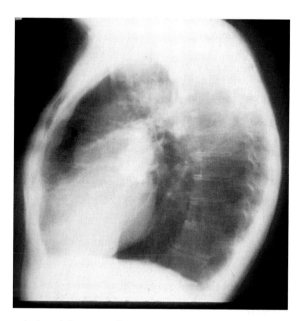

'Barrel-shaped chest'. Increased retrosternal air space. Note the flattened diaphragms.

Diaphragmatic rupture/hernia

Characteristics

- Results from direct blunt or penetrating trauma to the chest/abdomen.
- Difficult to diagnose. Complications often present late secondary to herniation of abdominal contents into the thoracic cavity. Visceral herniation may result in ischaemia, obstruction or perforation. Lung compression/collapse may be significant.
- More commonly affects the left side as liver is thought to protect the right.
- Postero-lateral radial tears are most commonly seen in blunt trauma.

Clinical features

- In the acute setting features tend to be obscured by other injuries.
- Examination may reveal tachypnoea, hypotension, absence of breath sounds or bowel sounds within the chest.
- With time (months to years), symptoms are often vague with abdominal discomfort relating to herniation of abdominal viscera.
- Symptoms similar to those of peptic ulceration, gall bladder disease, dysfunctional bowel syndromes and even ischaemic heart disease may be seen.
- Rarely the patient may present with a tension viscero-thorax mimicking a tension pneumothorax.
- Suspect in a patient with acute obstruction or unusual chest signs with a previous history of thoraco-abdominal trauma.

Radiological features

- In the acute phase, unless there is visceral herniation, sensitivity is poor for all imaging modalities.
- CXR:
  - Air filled or solid appearing viscus above the diaphragm. This may only be recognised following passage of an NG tube.
  - Other features include mediastinal shift away from the affected side, diaphragmatic elevation, apparent unilateral pleural thickening or suspicious areas of atelectasis.
- In the non-acute setting contrast studies may be useful.

Management

- ABCs.
- An NG tube may decompress the gastrointestinal tract.
- If perforation is suspected treat sepsis early.
- Discuss urgently with the surgical team.
- Planned elective surgery for late presentations.

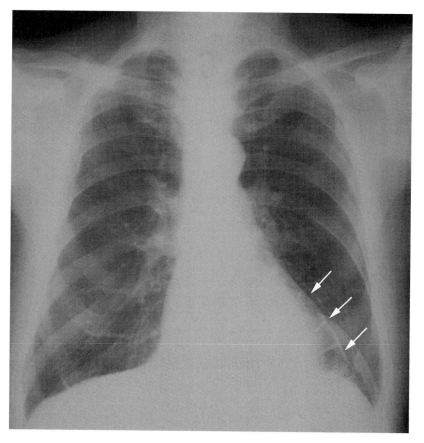

Late presentation of a diaphragmatic rupture. The arrows denote bowel which has herniated through a left diaphragmatic defect.

Flail chest

Characteristics

- Occurs when there is loss of continuity of a segment of chest wall with the rest of the thoracic cage.
- Usually traumatic with two or more ribs fractured in two or more places.
- Results in disruption of normal chest wall movements, and paradoxical movement may be seen.
- Always consider underlying lung injury (pulmonary contusion).
- The combination of pain, decreased or paradoxical chest wall movements and underlying lung contusion are likely to contribute to the patient's hypoxia.

Clinical features

- Dyspnoea
- Tachycardia
- Cyanosis
- Tachypnoea
- Hypotension
- Chest wall bruising $\pm$ palpable abnormal movement or rib crepitus
- The degree of hypoxia often depends on the severity of the underlying pulmonary contusion.

Radiological features

- Multiple rib fractures.
- Costochondral separation may not be evident.
- Air space shadowing may be seen with pulmonary contusions (often absent on initial films).

Management

- ABCs.
- In the absence of systemic hypotension judicious fluid replacement is required as the injured lung is susceptible to both under-resuscitation and fluid overload.
- Definitive treatment includes judicious fluid therapy, oxygenation and adequate analgesia to optimise ventilation/lung re-expansion.

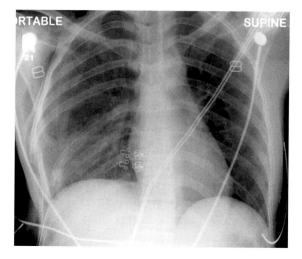

Right flail chest.

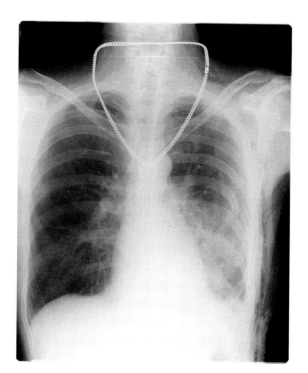

Left flail chest.

Foreign body – Inhaled foreign bodies

Characteristics

- Usually seen in children.
- Considered an emergency as it may result in complete upper airway obstruction.

Clinical features

- Spectrum from complete upper airway obstruction (distressed, agitated and choking child leading to unresponsiveness with associated pre-morbidity) to an asymptomatic child, or a child with a persistent cough.
- Auscultation of the chest may be normal. Monophonic wheeze is characteristic of large airway obstruction. Beware the localised absence of breath sounds.

Radiological features

- A radio-opaque foreign body may or may not be seen.
- Look for secondary signs, such as loss of volume, segmental collapse, consolidation or hyperinflation, as the foreign body acts as a ball valve.

Management

- If the child is coughing they should be encouraged.
- Do not intervene unless the child's cough becomes ineffective (quieter) or the child is losing consciousness. A spontaneous cough is more effective than assisting manoeuvres.
- Choking child procedure involves back blows, chest thrusts (same landmarks as for cardiac compression) and abdominal thrusts (omit in infants) repeated as a cycle (see below).
- If the choking child procedure fails the child may require laryngoscopy. Contact a senior anaesthetist and ENT surgeon urgently. Do not attempt this without the required experience, unless there is no option, as this may compromise the airway further.

Choking child algorithm

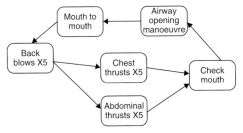

In an infant it is advised to avoid abdominal thrusts and thus alternate back blows with chest thrusts are suggested.

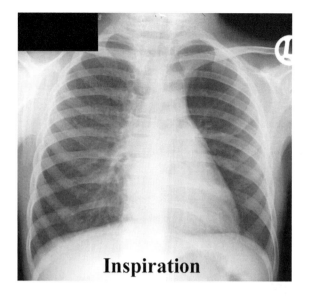

Inspiration

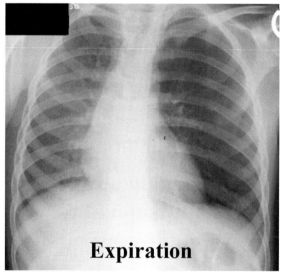

Expiration

'Ball valve' effect due to an inhaled foreign body. The air trapping is much more apparent on the expiratory scans.

Foreign body – Ingested foreign bodies

Characteristics

- Swallowed foreign bodies tend to lodge at sites of anatomical narrowing. These are at the level of cricopharyngeus, at the levels of the aortic arch and left main stem bronchus, and at the gastro-oesophageal junction.
- In children, cricopharyngeus is the most likely site of impaction. Once past this level, objects tend to pass through without hindrance. Impaction distal to this level should raise the possibility of pathological narrowing, such as a stricture.
- In adults foreign body ingestion is deliberate (self-harm), accidental (fish or chicken bones) or as the result of a diminished gag reflex.
- Complications result from the direct trauma caused by the foreign body, secondary pressure necrosis or during its' removal.

Clinical features

- Sensation of the presence of the foreign body.
- Features relating to complications, e.g. oesophageal perforation.

Radiological features

- A *lateral cervical soft tissue* radiograph may reveal a radio-opaque foreign body.
- Soft tissue swelling may be the only indicator of a radiolucent foreign body.
- A *water soluble contrast swallow* may demonstrate an intraluminal foreign body or outline a complication.

Management

- ABCs.
- Visualisation, both direct and indirect, with good lighting is useful and may allow removal of a visible foreign body.
- Refer patients who are symptomatic, and for whom an obvious cause cannot be seen and removed.
- Endoscopy allows definitive management.
- Beware of patients swallowing potentially dangerous items, such as button batteries (e.g. watch batteries) and sharp objects, such as razor blades!
- In a child, a CXR should be performed to demonstrate the site of the object. An AXR is required if the object is not seen within the chest to both confirm passage into the abdomen, and for transit monitoring if the object does not appear in the stool after 1–2 days.

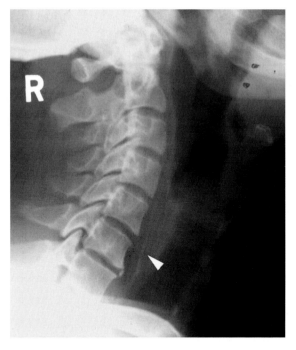

Fishbone (arrow) lodged in the hypopharynx anterior to C6.

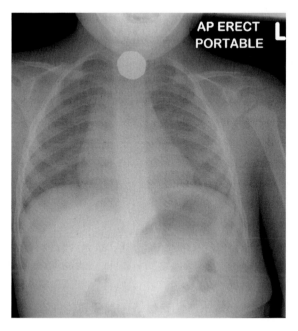

Swallowed metallic coin projected over the superior mediastinum.

Haemothorax

Characteristics

- Accumulation of blood within the pleural space following blunt or penetrating trauma.
- Commonly associated with a pneumothorax and other extrathoracic injuries.
- Haemorrhage usually occurs from the lung parenchyma, and is often self-limiting, rather than from a specific vessel injury. Intercostal and internal mammary vessels are more commonly injured than the hilar or great vessels.

Clinical features

- Depends mainly on the amount of blood lost.
- Varying degrees of hypovolaemic shock.
- Breath sounds – reduced or absent and/or dull to percussion.

Radiological features

- Erect CXR is more sensitive than a supine film.
    - Blunting of the costophrenic angles – seen with approximately 250 ml of blood.
    - General increased opacification of the hemithorax is seen on a supine film.

Management

- ABCs (with i.v. access prior to tube thoracostomy).
- Definitive management involves the placement of a large bore tube thoracostomy. This allows both re-expansion of lung as well as estimation of initial and ongoing blood loss. Airway control and circulatory volume support are essential alongside definitive treatment. A patient with initial drainage of 1500 mls or >200 mls/h are likely to require thoracotomy. Discuss with the thoracic team and be guided by the patient's physiological status.

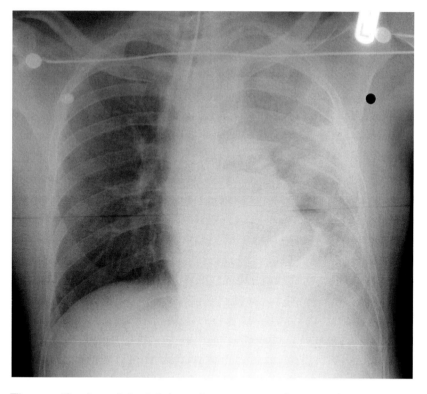

The opacification of the left hemithorax is secondary to a haemothorax.
This patient has a traumatic transaction of the aorta (see aortic rupture).

Oesophageal perforation/rupture

Characteristics

- Classically described following a forceful vomiting (*Boerhaave syndrome*).
- Commoner causes include – iatrogenic trauma, blunt/penetrating trauma, chemical injury, foreign body perforation, spontaneous rupture and post-operative breakdown.
- The oesophagus has no serosal covering and hence perforation allows direct access to the mediastinum.
- Perforation of the upper/cervical oesophagus allows access to the retropharygeal space.
- Perforation of the lower/mid-oesophagus tends to directly enter the mediastinum.
  - Inflammatory reaction causes contamination of the pleural space. This is facilitated by negative pleural pressure.

Clinical features

- Retrosternal pain is common. This is aggravated by swallowing or neck flexion. Radiation to the inter-scapular region. The pain is usually pro-gressive and may localise over time.
- Signs are often sparse and late, and relate to mediastinal air and pleural contamination. These include subcutaneous emphysema and a crunching sound on cardiac auscultation known as *Hamman's* crunch.
- Other signs secondary to a hydrothorax or an empyema may be present.
- A spontaneous pneumomediastinum may mimic an oesophageal rupture, but this tends to occur in the younger age group and often follows an extreme valsalva manoeuvre.
- As the inflammatory process progresses the patient's condition will deteri-orate with signs of sepsis and cardiopulmonary collapse.

Radiological features

- *CXR*: Classic signs are subcutaneous emphysema, pneumomediastinum, left sided pleural effusion, hydropneumothorax and mediastinal widening.
- *Cervical spine*: Lateral views may reveal retropharyngeal air.
- Pleural effusions, pulmonary infiltrates and a true mediastinal air–fluid level are not typically seen with a *spontaneous pneumomediastinum*.
- *Water soluble contrast studies* are of benefit to demonstrate perforations. If no perforation is seen a barium swallow will show better mucosal detail. These studies can be repeated over time.

Management

- ABCs.
- Suspect from the history. Time is of the essence.

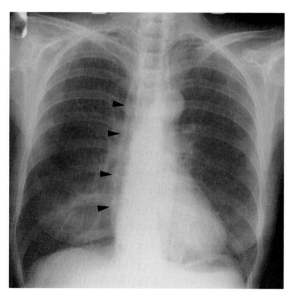

Oesophageal rupture. Air is seen outlining the right side of the mediastinum (arrowheads).

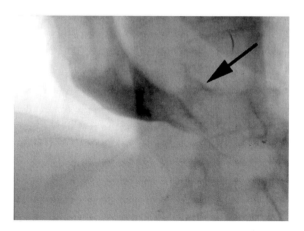

This is an inverted image from a water soluble swallow. This demonstrates the leak of contrast (arrow) from the distal third of the oesophagus.

- Give supplemental oxygen, analgesia, keep the patient nil by mouth, fluid replacement, start broad spectrum antibiotics and obtain a surgical consult. An NG tube can be carefully passed to decompress the stomach.
- Early surgical repair.

Pneumonia

Characteristics

- Incidence is increasing – due to an ageing population and the increased prevalence of immunosuppression.
- Types:
  - *Community acquired*: *Streptococcus* (>60%), *Haemophilus, Mycoplasma, Legionella* and *Chlamydia*. Generally low mortality unless admission required.
  - *Hospital acquired*: Increasingly Gram-negative infection. Higher mortality rate than community acquired pneumonias. Co-morbid factors are important.
- Organism virulence and load, host factors and early administration of appropriate therapy all contribute to outcome.
- Pneumonia should always be considered in the elderly, the immuno-compromised and in pyrexia of unknown origin (PUO).
- The prevalence of tuberculosis (TB) is increasing. *Suspect it!*

Clinical features

- Productive cough, dyspnoea, pleuritic chest pain, myalgia and haemo-ptysis may occur.
- In the immuno-suppressed patient *Pneumocystis* may present with profound hypoxia and little else on examination.
- The young patient may present with vague symptoms, such as headache, abdominal pain or even diarrhoea. Confusion may be the only sign in the elderly.
- Examination may reveal coarse inspiratory crepitations. Bronchial breathing with a dull percussion note is present in <25%.
- Poor prognostic signs include – age >60, respiratory rate >30, profound hypotension, acute confusion, urea >7 mmol/l and a markedly low or raised white cell count (WCC).

Radiological features

May lag behind clinical onset and remain after resolution!
- *Lobar pneumonia*: Opacification of a lobe; usually *Streptococcus*. Air bronchograms may be present.
- *Primary TB*: Right paratracheal (40%) and right hilar adenopathy (60%) with consolidation in the lower or mid-zones.
- *Post-primary TB*: Ill-defined consolidation in the apical segments which may cavitate.
- *Right middle and lower lobe pneumonia*: Loss of the right heart border and the right hemidiaphragm silhouette, respectively.
- *Lingular segment pneumonia*: Loss of the left heart border.
- *Left lower lobe consolidation*: Typically obliterates an arc of left hemi-diaphragm. Look 'through the heart' for loss of diaphragmatic outline.

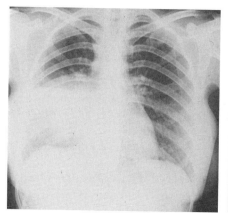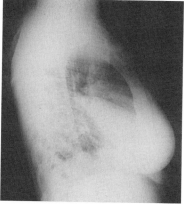

Right middle lobe pneumonia. Effacement of the right heart border. On the lateral view opacification of the middle lobe is seen between the horizontal and oblique fissures.

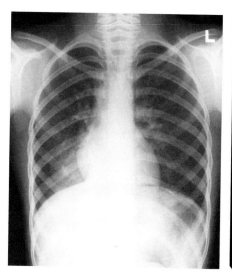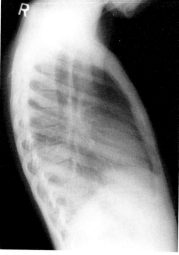

Right lower lobe pneumonia. Normally the retrocardiac and retrosternal air spaces should be of similar densities. However there is patchy opacification in the right lower zone which is seen in the retrocardiac airspace, secondary to consolidation.

Pneumonia (*continued*)

Management

- ABCs.
- Most patients can be discharged with appropriate oral antibiotics.
- Give advice regarding deep breathing and coughing.
- A NSAID may be of benefit in patients with pleuritic pain to enable deep breathing and coughing.
- Treat the unwell patient with high flow oxygen (remember the patient with chronic obstructive pulmonary disease (COPD) is often dependent on their hypoxic drive to stimulate respiration), i.v. fluids, i.v. antibiotics $\pm$ analgesia.

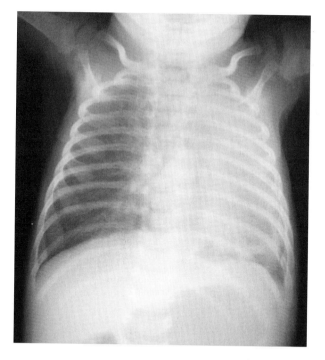

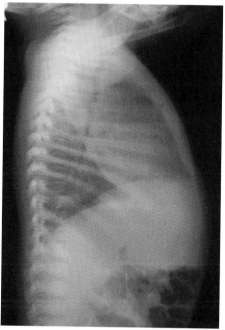

Left upper lobar pneumonia: note that the left hemidiaphragm is visible indicating that the pathology is not lower lobe. On the lateral view, extensive opacity is seen anterior to the oblique fissure in the upper lobe.

Pneumothorax

Characteristics

- Accumulation of air within the pleural cavity.
- A common complication of chest trauma (15–40%).
- Divided into three categories:
    (i) *Simple*: No communication with the atmosphere or mediastinum. No mid-line shift.
    (ii) *Communicating*: Associated with chest wall defect.
    (iii) *Tension*: Progressive accumulation of air under pressure within the pleural cavity; leading to mediastinal shift with compression of the contra-lateral lung and great vessels.

Clinical features

- Chest pain and shortness of breath are common.
- Variable spectrum ranging from acutely unwell, with cyanosis and tachypnoea, to the relatively asymptomatic patient.
- Signs and symptoms do not necessarily correlate well with the degree of associated lung collapse.
    - Signs of a tension pneumothorax include:
        - Tachycardia
        - Jugulo-venous distension
        - Absent breaths sounds
        - Hyper-resonance to percussion
        - Tracheal and cardiac impulse displacement away from the affected side
        - The patient may be acutely unwell with signs of cardio-respiratory distress.

Radiological features

- *Simple*: Visceral pleural edge visible. Loss of volume on the affected side (e.g. raised hemidiaphragm). A small pneumothorax may not be visualised on a standard inspiratory film. A expiratory film may be of benefit.
- *Tension*: THIS IS A CLINICAL AND NOT A RADIOLOGICAL DIAGNOSIS! Associated mediastinal shift to the opposite side is seen.

Management

- ABCs.
- *Simple*: Depends on size and clinical picture.
    (i) Conservative treatment with follow-up CXR.
    (ii) Aspiration using a three-way tap may be adequate.
    (iii) Definitive management – tube thoracostomy.
- *Tension*
    (iv) Needle thoracostomy with a 14/16 g cannula in the 2nd intercostal space (mid-clavicular line).

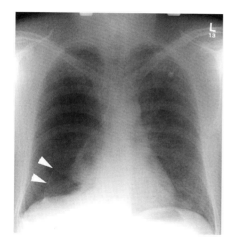

Simple pneumothorax: the edge of the right lung is clearly seen (arrows) devoid of peripheral lung markings. No mediastinal shift occurs.

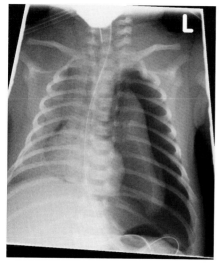

Iatrogenic tension pneumothorax. This is secondary to the high intra-thoracic pressures generated during ventilation resulting in rupture of a pleural bleb. There is progressive mediastinal shift to the right.

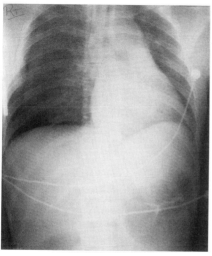

Traumatic tension pneumothorax. Right sided rib fractures and pneumothorax with mediastinal shift to the left.

Rib/sternal fracture

Characteristics

- Usually following direct trauma. May be pathological.
- Suspect with localised pain and tenderness which may be aggravated by deep inspiration or coughing.
- Consider associated injuries:
  - *Clavicle/1st or 2nd rib fractures* suggest or indicate a significant force, often associated with great vessel, tracheo-bronchial or spinal injury.
  - *Sterno-clavicular dislocation*, posterior (rarer) associated with increased risk of major visceral damage.
  - *Sternal injuries* may be associated with myocardial contusion.
  - With *lower rib fractures*, abdominal visceral injury, such as liver, spleen or kidney, may occur.

Clinical features

- Pain with limitation of inspiration.
- Often related to complications from any associated injury, e.g. cardiac dysrhythmias or splenic rupture.

Radiological features

- A CXR/lateral sternal view are performed to assess for both complications and to identify any underlying fracture.
- Signs of secondary complications may be evident – pneumothorax, haemothorax, pulmonary contusion, etc.

Management

- ABCs.
- Simple rib or sternal fractures with a normal electrocardiogram (ECG) and CXR (no secondary complications) – the patient can usually be discharged with respiratory advice and good analgesia; non-steroidal analgesia in combination with other analgesia is usually effective unless contra-indicated.
- If there are CXR or ECG changes refer for observation.

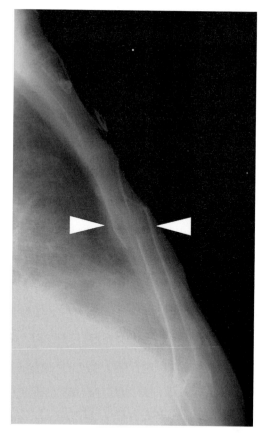

Sternal fracture.

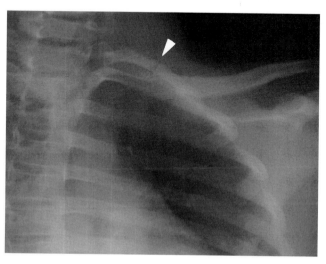

Fracture of the left first rib. This injury requires significant force and is associated with an increased incidence of neurovascular injury, particularly the subclavian vein.

Abdominal aortic aneurysms

Characteristics

- Defined as permanent localised dilatation of an artery affecting all layers of the vessel wall.
- Can develop in any part of the aorta but are most commonly seen below the level of the renal arteries.
- The aorta is larger in men and increases in size with age. A diameter of >3 cm is generally recognised as abnormal.
- May result from a specific cause, such as trauma, infection or inflammation. Most commonly accepted aetiology is atherosclerosis.
- Rare before the age of 50. Commoner in elderly men.
- Enlarge by approximately 0.2–0.5 cm/year.
- The risk of rupture increases with size of the aneurysm.

Clinical features

- Most aneurysms are discovered incidentally.
- May present secondary to embolic phenomena, be symptomatic from compression of adjacent structures or present with a classical rupture.
- A classical rupture presents with the triad of pain (often back pain), a pulsatile mass and hypotension. Beware as the patient may have none of the aforementioned!
- Duration of symptoms is often variable with some describing weeks of symptoms.
- Most rupture into the retroperitoneum, but can occasionally present as a fistula into adjacent bowel or into the vena cava.

Radiological features

- *Abdominal X-ray (AXR)*: Look for curvilinear 'egg shell' type calcification on the AXR, or evidence of a paravertebral soft tissue mass. A lateral film can provide additional information. Rarely vertebral body erosion may be seen with long standing aneurysms. With rupture, loss of the psoas outline may be seen.
- *Ultrasound (US)* can accurately determine size. Limited use in assessing rupture.
- *CT* is accurate in assessing aneurysm rupture as well as visualising adjacent structures.
- *CT* is also used to plan elective surgery.

Management

- ABCs.
- The patient with a ruptured aneurysm is unstable until surgical cross clamping of the proximal aorta at surgery has occurred.
- Suspect the diagnosis and involve the surgical team early, whist carefully resuscitating. The degree of volume resuscitation remains controversial. The aim is not to extend the haemorrhage whilst maintaining end-organ perfusion.

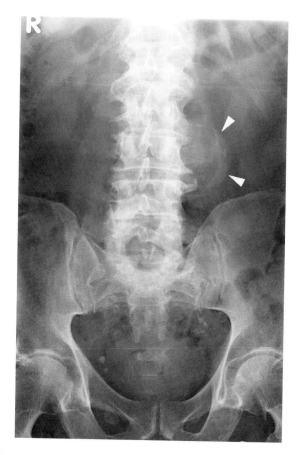

Calcification in the left lateral wall of an aortic aneurysm (arrowheads).

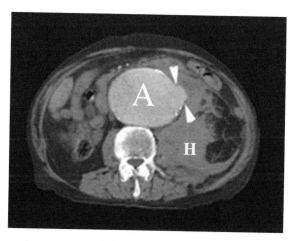

Ruptured aortic aneurysm. The arrowheads denote the breach in the wall of the aneurysm (A), with extensive associated retroperitoneal haemorrhage (H).

Appendicitis

Characteristics

- Relatively common condition seen in the 5–20 age group.
- Aetiology remains unknown. Probably related to luminal obstruction either by intraluminal or mural pathology.
- The inflammatory process will commonly result in localised peritonitis. Abscess formation and disseminated peritonitis can complicate.
- Beware in the elderly as appendicitis may occur and be missed.

Clinical features

- The patient classically presents with a history of central abdominal pain that localises to the right iliac fossa.
- Pyrexia, malaise, nausea and anorexia are common complaints.
- Atypical presentations with dysuria, frequency, bloating or diarrhoea do occur.
- On examination most will have localised tenderness with guarding. Rebound is an indicator of localised peritoneal inflammation.
- Right lower abdominal pain on palpation of the left lower quadrant is termed Rovsing's sign.
- Pain on passive extension of the right hip is a non-specific sign.

Radiological features

- *AXR*: Look for a calcified appendicolith in the right lower quadrant (RLQ). Other indicators include free air; small bowel ileus; extra-luminal gas; caecal wall thickening; loss of pelvis fat planes around the bladder suggests pelvic free fluid; loss of the properitoneal fat line; psoas line distortion and abrupt cut-off of the normal gaseous pattern at the hepatic flexure due to colonic spasm.
- *US*: Suggestive features include an obstructing appendicolith – a blind ending non-peristaltic, non-compressible tubular structure and prominent vasculature within the meso-appendix; wall thickness should be <2 mm in a normal appendix or <6 mm in total diameter.
- *CT*: Sensitive and specific investigation. Not routine due to radiation dose. Luminal distension with a thickened enhancing wall ± an appendicolith. Local inflammation shows as linear streaking in the adjacent fat. Abscesses may be present.
- *Contrast investigations*: Occasionally picked up coincidently. Suggested by non-filling or localised mucosal oedema within the caecal pole.

Management

- Fluid resuscitate, analgesia and anti-emetics if required. Urinalysis and routine bloods. Do a pregnancy test in females of child-bearing age. Discuss with the surgical team.

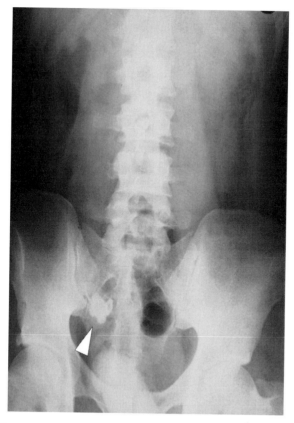

Large calcified appendicolith (arrowhead).

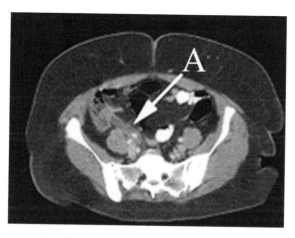

Inflammed appendix (A) with an intraluminal appendicolith at the tip.

Intussusception

Characteristics

- Occurs when a segment of intestine prolapses into the lumen of adjacent intestine.
- Regarded as a paediatric disease, but does occur in adults.
- Commonest cause of bowel obstruction in young children and infants (3 months–5 years). Rare under the age of 1 month.
- Occurs in approximately 1 in 2000 below the age of 15.
- Increased incidence seen in siblings of affected children.
- Less than 10% of children have an identifiable lead point, such as a Meckel's diverticulum or lymphoid hyperplasia.
- In adults a lead point is found in the majority (nasogastric (NG) tube, foreign body, tumour, etc.).

Clinical features

- Severe colicky abdominal pain with associated vomiting.
- Young children will often draw their knees up to their chest and can be very lethargic. In between attacks, the child may appear relatively well.
- In a classical presentation a sausage-shaped mass will be felt in the abdomen and the child will oblige by passing 'red currant' stools.

Radiological features

- *AXR*: On a plain film look for a soft tissue mass sometimes with evidence of proximal bowel obstruction.
- *Contrast studies* will show a coiled-spring appearance. A beak-like narrowing can be seen with antegrade studies.
- *US* is the gold standard and is close to 100% sensitive. Signs described include a target or bull's eye appearance on transverse scanning. A sandwich appearance is described on longitudinal scanning. Colour Doppler can be used to assess vascular supply.
- *CT*: Multiple concentric rings are diagnostic.

Management

- Discuss with the surgical team.
- Hydrostatic or pneumatic reduction is the recommended treatment. Surgical reduction is indicated if there are signs of peritonism, free air or following failed hydrostatic/pneumatic reduction.

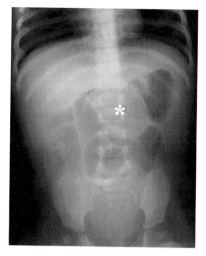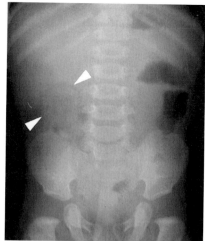

Two examples of intussusception seen as a soft tissue mass.

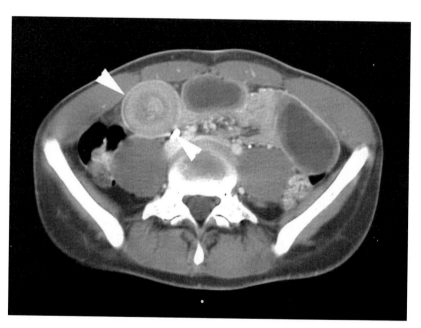

Cross sectional image of a jejunal intussusception. Note the obstructed proximal small bowel.

Ischaemic colitis

Characteristics

- More than 90% of cases occur in the elderly.
- Although the major mesenteric vessels are usually patent, reduced blood flow within the inferior mesenteric artery territory leads to ischaemia of the mucosa and submucosa.
- Can be precipitated by a variety of causes including bowel obstruction, emboli or thrombosis. Distant causes, such as shock and congestive heart failure, can also cause ischaemia. Not an uncommon complication of aneurysm repair.
- Has also been described secondary to vasoconstrictive drugs, such as cocaine.
- Tends to affect the left side of the colon with the splenic flexure and sigmoid being the commonest areas affected. The rectum is usually spared.

Clinical features

- Classically presents as severe lower abdominal pain followed by bloody diarrhoea.
- Three distinct subgroups have been described:
  1. *Gangrenous*: Vascular supply completely interrupted leading to transmural infarction. Perforation and peritonitis result.
  2. *Stricturing*: Impaired vascular supply leads to mucosal and submucosal ischaemia. Ulceration occurs with healing by fibrosis and results in stenosis.
  3. *Transient*: Reversible vascular impairment leads to mucosal sloughing with subsequent regeneration.

Radiological features

- *AXR*: Plain films tend to be normal. Marginal thumb printing on the mesenteric side may be seen related to pericolic fat inflammation.
- A *barium enema* will show mucosal thumb printing related to submucosal haemorrhage and oedema. Markedly oedematous mucosal folds show as transverse ridges. Shallow ulceration can be seen but deep ulceration is a late sign.
- *CT* may demonstrate thickening of the affected segment. Clot within the mesenteric vessels is sometimes seen. Air within the bowel wall or within the venous system is a late sign.
- *US* may show wall thickening but vascular assessment with Doppler studies is usually limited.

Management

- Fluid resuscitate and consult the surgical team. Non-occlusive ischaemic colitis is generally best managed conservatively.

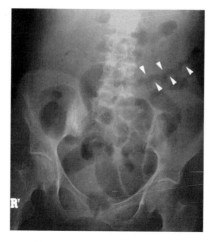

Mucosal 'thumb printing' in an ischaemic segment.

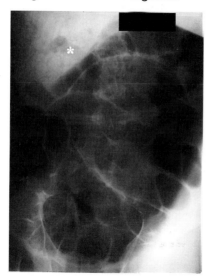

Necrotic perforated large bowel. Air is seen in the portal vein (*).

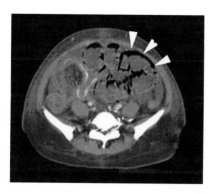

Air seen within the bowel wall: a CT feature of late ischaemia.

Obstruction – Large bowel obstruction

Characteristics

- Less commonly seen than small bowel obstruction.
- In western societies, the commonest cause of mechanical obstruction is malignancy.
- Other causes include diverticulitis and inflammatory, ischaemic or radiation induced colitis. Paralytic ileus and pseudo-obstruction are also common.
- As expected, obstruction is commoner in the elderly.
- If the ileocaecal valve is patent a closed loop obstruction occurs leading to vascular compromise and ischaemia. Perforation results if the obstruction is not relieved.

Clinical features

- Crampy lower abdominal pain often develops insidiously and is associated with constipation.
- Abdominal distension tends to be more marked than in small bowel obstruction. Vomiting is a late sign in large bowel obstruction and occurs if the ileocaecal valve is incompetent.
- Localised pain, with signs of peritonism, is suggestive of ischaemia or per-foration. The caecum is the most likely site to perforate.

Radiological features

- *AXR*: Plain abdominal films are often diagnostic. The large bowel is seen to be dilated peripherally ('picture frame' appearance). Note the haustral pattern does not fully traverse the colon as compared to small bowel valvulae conniventes.
- Distended small bowel loops seen with an incompetent ileocaecal valve.
- Caecal distension >8 cm increases the likelihood of caecal perforation.
- An erect chest radiograph (CXR) or lateral decubitus film should be performed if perforation is suspected.
- Contrast studies can be helpful to delineate the site of obstruction.

Management

- Fluid resuscitate and correct electrolyte disturbances.
- Gastric and intestinal decompression with a NG tube is indicated.
- Broad spectrum antibiotics.
- Consult the surgical team.

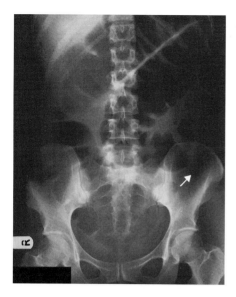

Large bowel obstruction. A transition point is seen in the region of the sigmoid colon.

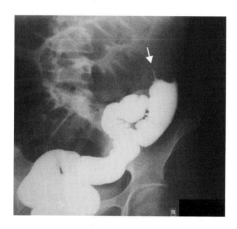

The instant enema on the same patient demonstrate the obstructing lesion.

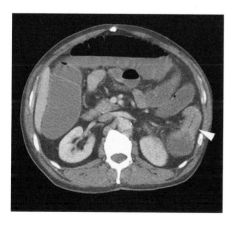

Annular soft tissue mass obstructing the mid-descending colon.

Obstruction – Small bowel obstruction

Characteristics

- Classified as *dynamic* or *adynamic*.
- With dynamic obstruction the bowel tries to overcome a physical barrier. Causes can be divided into intraluminal (neoplasm, intussusception and foreign body); mural (neoplasm and stricture) or extrinsic (adhesions, hernia, volvulus and neoplasm).
- With adynamic obstruction the bowel peristalsis is decreased or absent. Typically seen in response to inflammation, e.g. peritonitis or post-laparotomy.
- *Pseudo-obstruction* often has the symptoms and signs of obstruction without a cause being found. Associated with a variety of medical conditions.

Clinical features (dynamic)

- Crampy abdominal pain, distension and vomiting are common. The pain is often localised poorly in the epigastrium or periumbilical region. Flatus and stool passage are typically preserved until late in small bowel obstruction.
- In general, the more proximal the obstruction, the shorter the presentation.
- Look for distension, scars and herniae. The abdomen may be tympanic to percussion with increased 'tinkling' bowel sounds.
- Marked tenderness suggests complicated obstruction and signs of bowel ischaemia should be looked for. Strangulated bowel is difficult to diagnose from examination alone.

Radiological features

- *AXR*: Small bowel can be differentiated from large by the valvulae conniventes which cross the bowel completely, as compared to the haustral pattern of large bowel. Another indicator is the site (central vs. marginal). Look for dilated loops of centrally located bowel lying adjacent to each other (step ladder appearance) in distal obstruction. Compare diameter of adjacent small bowel loops (<3 cm is normal). Colonic gas is often sparse or absent. On the erect film multiple (>3) air–fluid levels are suggestive. Beware the patient with grossly fluid-filled bowel as this may be missed.
- *Contrast studies*: Small bowel enema is more sensitive than a follow through.
- *CT*: Useful in assessing both the level of obstruction and for the presence of extra-luminal pathology.

Management

- Fluid resuscitation, analgesia, bowel decompression with an NG tube and referral to the surgical team. Consider antibiotics if complication suspected.

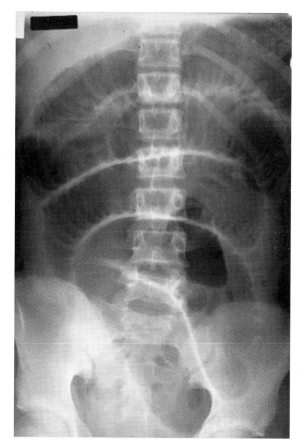

Classic small bowel obstruction: valvulae conniventes clearly demonstrated. Note that the hernial orifices have not been included on the radiograph.

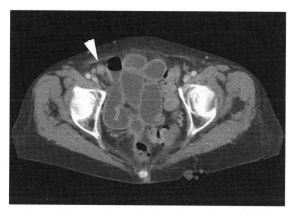

Femoral hernia: the arrowhead denotes a collapsed loop of small bowel in the femoral canal with obstructed proximal small bowel.

Perforation

Characteristics

- Perforation of an air containing hollow viscus, such as duodenum or sigmoid colon diverticulum, will result in free intraperitoneal air.
- Other common sites for perforation include the appendix in acute appendicitis and the colon secondary to mechanical large bowel obstruction or a toxic megacolon.
- Small bowel perforation is seen with trauma, foreign body ingestion and with infiltrative disorders, such as lymphoma.
- The age of the patient and a thorough history will often pinpoint the site of a viscus perforation.

Clinical features

- Pain is generally common to all perforations. Initially localised it can become generalised as peritonitis sets in.
- The site of pain can indicate the viscus involved. Upper abdominal pain suggests stomach or duodenum, whereas lower abdominal pain suggests colon.
- Tenderness and guarding will follow a similar pattern, initially localised then generalised.
- Liver dullness will be reduced if air is interspaced between the liver and anterior abdominal wall.
- Bowel sounds are reduced or absent with generalised peritonitis.
- Beware the elderly patient with vague symptoms and signs.

Radiological features

- *CXR*: An *erect* CXR is a sensitive method of demonstrating free sub-diaphragmatic air. Volumes as small as 1–2 ml of free air may be detected. Beware the supine patient elevated just prior to obtaining the erect film.
- *AXR*: A *lateral decubitus* film (usually right side up) can be of use if an erect film cannot be obtained. Air will then outline the lateral edge of the liver. When there is free air within the abdomen the bowel becomes clearly delineated due to the presence of air on both sides of the bowel wall. This is termed *Riggler's* sign.
- Look for outlining of other intra-abdominal structures not usually well seen. These include the diaphragmatic muscle slips, lateral and medial umbilical ligaments, falciform ligament and the liver.
- Pitfalls include contained gas mistaken for free air. Chiliaditi syndrome describes colonic gas seen interposed between liver and the abdominal wall. Diverticular, herniae, sub-diaphragmatic abscesses and chest pathology can all be mistaken for free air.

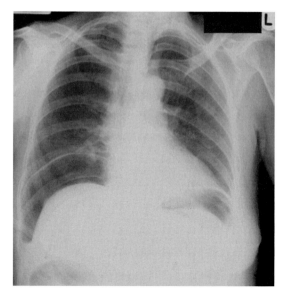

Pneumoperitoneum: free air under both hemidiaphragms.

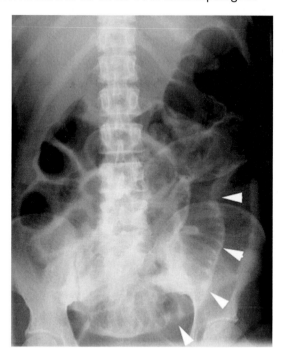

Pneumoperitoneum: note the Riggler's sign (arrowheads).

Management

- Most of the above conditions will require surgical management.
- Provide adequate analgesia, fluid resuscitate and refer. Obtain appropriate blood and radiological investigations.

Renal/ureteric calculi

Characteristics

- Commonest disorder of the urinary tract.
- Five to ten per cent of the population will develop renal tract calculi.
- Male predominance, occurring commonly in 20–50-year olds.
- There is a family tendency towards stone formation. Recurrent attacks are commoner than a single episode.
- The majority of stones are composed of calcium oxalate (also the most radio-opaque).

Clinical features

- Renal colic classically presents as severe colicky loin to groin pain that builds to a crescendo.
- The patient will often appear restless and agitated with the pain.
- Nausea and vomiting are commonly associated.
- Commoner during the night or early morning.
- Urgency, frequency and dysuria also commonly occur.

Radiological features

- *Kidney, ureter, bladder (KUB)*: This will show >70% of calculi; thus around 30% are not visible. Carefully examine adjacent to the tips of the transverse processes, the sacro-iliac joint and pelvic cavity for opacities suggestive of calculi (irregular shape). Phleboliths tend to be spherical with a lucent centre. Calcified lymph nodes may also be mistaken.
- *Intravenous pyelogram (IVP)*: A 5 minute and 20 minute post-micturition films should be obtained. Look for a delayed nephrogram, pelvicalyceal blunting, hydronephrosis and/or a standing column of contrast in the ureter. Delayed films can be of benefit.
- *CT*: Sensitive and specific test.

Management

- Adequate analgesia is essential. Non-steroidal anti-inflammatory drugs (NSAIDs) are effective pain relievers and also help reduce ureteric spasm. Beware the frequent attendee requesting pethidine.
- Sepsis or obstruction is an indication for admission. Otherwise the patient can be discharged with advice and analgesia for outpatient follow-up.

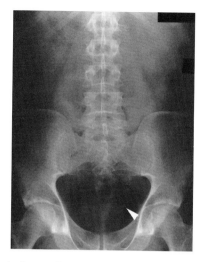
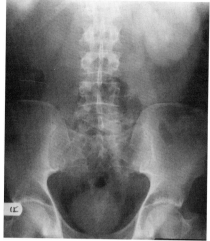

Left renal tract obstruction secondary to a left vesico-ureteric calculus (arrowhead).

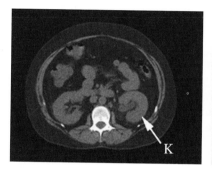
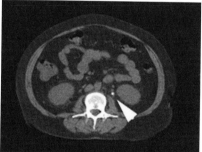

Unenhanced renal tract CT. This demonstrates an obstructing calculus in the upper third of the left ureter.

Sigmoid volvulus

Characteristics

- Occurs when the sigmoid colon rotates causing a closed loop obstruction. Vascular compromise may occur. Predisposed in patients with a redundant sigmoid loop and a narrow mesentery.
- Likely to be related to chronic severe constipation.
- Occurs in the elderly and in patients with severe psychiatric or neurological diseases.

Clinical features

- Patients will often present late and provide a poor history. Suspect in the elderly or senile patients with obstruction.
- Crampy lower abdominal pain with associated distension is common.
- Absolute constipation and tenesmus (secondary to rectal traction).
- Similar episodes in the past are often described, often self-terminating following passage of a motion.
- Beware signs of sepsis as these indicate likely gangrene. Perforation is uncommon.

Radiological features

- On *plain abdominal films*, look for a loop of large bowel extending upwards from the pelvis. Described as a 'coffee bean' appearance.
- *Barium studies* can be performed as long as gangrene is not suspected. The barium characteristically tapers in the shape of a bird's beak.
- A whirled pattern has been described on CT. This is formed from the twisted afferent and efferent loops of bowel.

Management

- Fluid resuscitate and correct electrolyte disturbances.
- Gastric and intestinal decompression with a NG tube is indicated.
- Broad spectrum antibiotics.
- Consult the surgical team as early decompression via a sigmoidoscope and flatus tube may prevent ischaemic complications.
- Surgical resection necessary if conservative decompression fails.

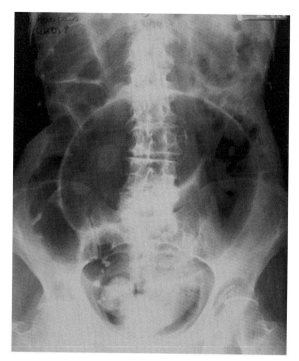

Classic sigmoid volvulus: 'Coffee bean' sign.

Toxic megacolon (fulminant colitis)

Characteristics

- This usually develops secondary to a fulminant colitis (usually ulcerative colitis).
- Fulminant colitis occurs in roughly 10% of patients with ulcerative colitis. Of these only a proportion will develop toxic megacolon.
- Usually occurs during the initial presentation of acute fulminant colitis.
- Can be precipitated by enema use, overuse of antidiarrhoeal agents or by barium enema investigation.

Clinical features

- Features include abdominal pain with distension which is progressive.
- On examination the abdomen is tender. Signs of sepsis including fever, rigors and tachycardia are often present.
- A recent history may reveal recent poor control of the underlying ulcerative colitis.
- Approximately 25% of patients with toxic megacolon will develop a perforation. This is suggested clinically by localised pain progressing to generalised peritonitis with deterioration in the clinical picture.

Radiological features

- *Best seen on plain AXR.* The transverse colon (TC) is most commonly affected. Radiographic signs suggestive include:
  - Size >8 cm. The upper limit of normal is 6 cm.
  - Pseudopolyps represent islands of mucosa with surrounding mucosal loss.
  - Pneumotosis coli – air within the bowel wall secondary to necrosis.
  - Free air secondary to perforation. A lateral decubitus film may be helpful.
  - Loss of the normal haustral pattern.
- *CT:* Distended colon with a nodular thin wall. Intramural air and fluid collection.
- Barium enema is *contraindicated*.

Management

- Toxic megacolon is an indication for surgery. Fluid resuscitate the patient and liaise with the surgical team early.

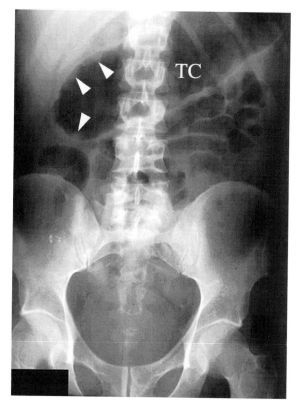

Toxic megacolon: oedematous mucosal 'islands' (arrowheads) in an inflamed TC.

Trauma – Blunt abdominal trauma

Characteristics

- Commonly seen after road traffic accidents.
- Often difficult to assess due to multi-system injury.
- Injuries tend to occur secondary to the following three mechanisms:
    (i) *Intra-abdominal pressure rises*: Leading to hollow organ injury.
    (ii) *Compression*: Viscera compressed between the anterior abdominal wall and the vertebral column/posterior thoracic cage. Spleen and liver are commonly injured.
    (iii) *Shear forces*: Result in pedicle injuries. Lacerations are also commonly seen at sites of fixed attachment.
- Beware of lower thoracic injuries, such as those produced with conventional seat belts; there are also associated liver/splenic injuries.
- Lap belts can produce mesenteric/bowel tears and contusions. May cause perforation secondary to a sudden rise in intraluminal pressure.

Clinical features

- A spectrum of relatively benign appearing features to the collapsed hypotensive patient may be seen.
- The patient will often complain of pain that may or may not be well localised.
- Involuntary guarding suggests peritoneal irritation. Rebound indicates established peritoneal irritation. Frequent reassessment by the same examiner is recommended to assess for changes.
- Examination is not as reliable in the compromised patient.
- Look for characteristic bruising that may suggest a visceral injury. When appropriate, adjuncts, such as NG and bladder intubation, can provide additional information.

Radiological features

- *Plain films*: Rib, transverse process, vertebral body and pelvic fractures are important as these indicate potential injury to adjacent structures. Fluid within the abdomen can be seen to displace gaseous structures, such as the ascending/descending colon medially. Small bowel gravitates centrally in the supine fluid-filled abdomen. Free air will gravitate and thus will be seen under the diaphragm in the erect film. On the supine film look for air along peritoneal attachments, such as the falciform ligament. Retroperitoneal air will outline adjacent structures, such as kidney and duodenum. A lateral decubitus film can be helpful.
- *US*: A quick non-invasive repeatable investigation which is sensitive for free fluid (>100 ml) within the abdomen. Focused examination of the splenorenal recess, Morrison's pouch and the pouch of Douglas ± paracolic regions is sensitive for free fluid. This examination has the advantage of not being restricted to the radiologist. Useful also to assess the diaphragm.

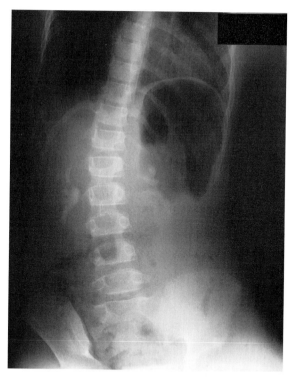

Closed blunt renal trauma. There is asymmetry between the two renal outlines. The left renal outline and opacification of the left pelvicalyceal system (PC) is distorted. In addition, there is scoliosis of the thoracolumbar region, concave to the side of injury with an associated localised ileus at the splenic flexure. The right PC system appears normal.

Trauma (continued)

- *CT*: Very useful in blunt abdominal trauma. Can define visceral injury as well as free haemorrhage. Can be extended to examine above and below the diaphragm. More useful than US and Diagnostic peritoneal lavage (DPL) to assess retroperitoneal injury. Can be repeated to follow up an injury. Less sensitive for small bowel, pancreatic and diaphragmatic injuries.
- *Contrast studies*: Useful if there is suspected oesophageal, gastric or duodenal perforation.
- *Angiography*: Used in selected patients.

Management

- ABCs.
- Involve the surgeon early. Indications for a laparotomy with blunt abdominal trauma include recurrent hypotension despite resuscitation, free air, peritonitis and diaphragmatic rupture.

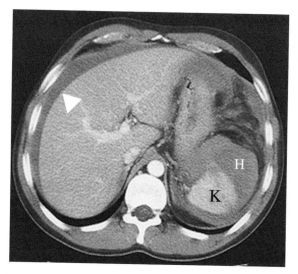

Blunt renal trauma. Large peri-renal haematoma (H) and additional free peritoneal blood (arrowhead). K: kidney.

Trauma – Penetrating abdominal trauma

Characteristics

- Increasing in incidence.
- Stab and gunshot wounds account for the majority of injuries. Although stab injuries account for approximately 80% of injuries, the vast majority of deaths are firearm related.
- Liver, spleen, small and large bowel, and stomach are commonly involved.
- Mortality is related to degree of hypovolaemia and the number of organs injured.

Clinical features

- Features relate to the type, character and number of penetrating injuries.
- Obtain a history from witnesses, paramedics, patient, etc.
- As with blunt trauma, serial examinations should be carried out by the same person (preferably the surgeon on call).
- Beware the patient with lower chest, back and flank injuries as a retroperitoneal injury may not be apparent.

Radiological features

- Investigations should not delay management decisions. Should only be performed if an immediate laparotomy is not indicated.
- *Plain films*: Can reveal free intra-abdominal air or help to localise a radio-opaque foreign body.
- *US*: See blunt trauma. In penetrating trauma US can be used to assess the pericardial space for a collection. Has also been used to assess direction and depth of a penetrating tract.
- *CT*: See blunt trauma. Commonly not performed in cases of penetrating trauma as a clear indication for laparotomy is often present. Indicators of hypovolaemia have been described on CT; these should be correlated with clinical signs and do not replace repeated biophysical readings:
  - Inferior vena cava (IVC) flattening/collapse.
  - Poorly enhanced small spleen.
  - Intense vascular constriction indicated by small aorta and mesenteric arteries.

Management

- ABCs.
- Frequently reassess above. Ensure adequate fluid resuscitation in order to maximise end-organ perfusion and oxygenation.
- Involve the on-call surgeon early as careful physical assessment and reassessment are vital.

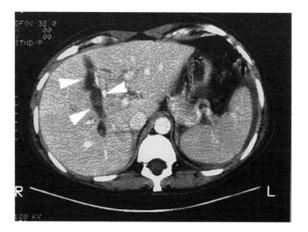

Large liver laceration.

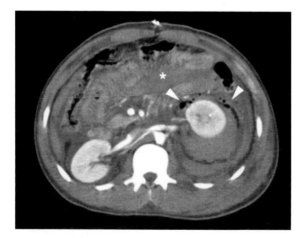

Peri-nephric haematoma with small pockets of contained air (arrowheads).

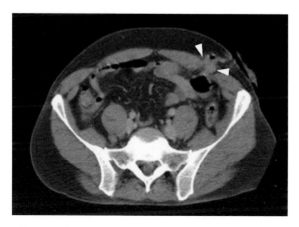

Herniation of bowel (arrowheads) following a stab injury.

UPPER LIMB

Acromio-clavicular joint injury

Characteristics

- Mechanism of injury commonly involves a blow to the point of the shoulder with the arm adducted. Contact sports are often involved.
- The acromio-clavicular (AC) ligaments rupture first followed by the coraco-clavicular ligaments and the muscular attachments of deltoid and trapezius.
- With a fall onto the outstretched hand, only the AC ligaments will be involved.
- Classified as follows:
  - *Sprain of ligaments*: Anatomical relationships preserved.
  - *Subluxation*: Rupture of the AC ligaments. The distal clavicle rides upwards, usually by less than half its width. Coraco-clavicular ligaments intact.
  - *Dislocation*: Rupture of the AC and coraco-clavicular ligaments. Trapezius and deltoid insertions avulsed. The coraco-clavicular distance is greatly increased as the clavicle rides upwards.
- Other classifications are used, such as the six grade Rockwood classification.

Clinical features

- Suspect from the history and ask the patient to point the site of pain.
- Examine the patient standing as this may allow asymmetry to be seen.
- With minor sprains, the patient will often complain of very localised pain and tenderness but a full range of movement is often possible.
- As the severity of sprain progresses the functional loss is more pronounced with a clinical deformity obvious.

Radiological features

- Recommended views include AP, 15 degree cephalic tilt and axial views.
- Specific AC joint views should be specified as the exposure is different from shoulder views.
- In the normal patient, the inferior surfaces of the acromion and clavicle are aligned.
- *Grade I* are radiographically normal. *Grade II* show widening of the joint with upward displacement of the clavicle. *Grade III* have a widened coraco-clavicular space (>13 mm or a difference of >5 mm between the two sides) and complete disruption of the AC joint (should be <8 mm).
- Stress views were commonly requested but cannot be recommended due to the discomfort caused and the high rate of false negatives seen from muscular spasm.

Management

- ABCs.
- *Grade I*: Analgesia and broad arm sling for comfort.

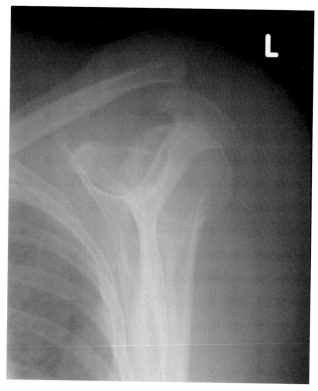

Acromio-clavicular joint dislocation.

- *Grade II*: As above but adequate follow-up recommended.
- *Grade III*: Adequate analgesia and broad arm sling. Controversy exists as to the best management of these cases, i.e. surgical vs. non-operative. Early orthopaedic referral is recommended (<72 hours).

Carpal dislocation (including lunate and perilunate dislocations)

Characteristics

- Generally occur following a fall onto the wrist/hand.
- Spectrum of injuries produced by wrist hyperextension, ulnar deviation and intercarpal supination.
- Classified into four categories:
  1. *Scapholunate dislocation*
  2. *Perilunate dislocation*
  3. *Perilunate dislocation with associated triquetral dislocation* (mid-carpal)
  4. *Lunate dislocation.*

Clinical features

- Patients will often complain of pain and swelling.
- Movement at the wrist will be limited.
- Localised tenderness especially in the scapholunate region.

Radiological features

- Postero-anterior (PA) and lateral views essential.
- Comparison with the opposite side often helpful.
- On the lateral view look at the relationship between the distal radius, lunate and capitate (often described as saucer, cup and apple).
- With *scapholunate dislocations*, there is an increased (>3 mm) gap between the scaphoid and the lunate on the AP view. This is described as the Terry Thomas sign after the aforementioned comedian's front teeth!
- With *perilunate dislocations*, the capitate is dislocated dorsally in relation to the lunate. The alignment of lunate and distal radius (saucer and cup) appears normal.
- In *mid-carpal dislocations*, appearances are similar to above except the triquetrum is dislocated. This is best seen on the PA view as it overlaps the lunate or hamate.
- With *lunate dislocations* the lunate dislocates forwards, i.e. the 'cup tips forwards spilling its contents' on the lateral view. The capitate remains aligned in relation to the radius. On the AP view, the lunate has a characteristic triangular appearance due to volar tilt.

Management

- ABCs.
- Analgesia and consult the orthopaedic team as these injuries often require open reduction and ligamentous repair.

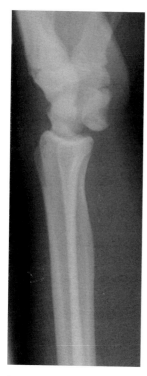

Lunate dislocation.

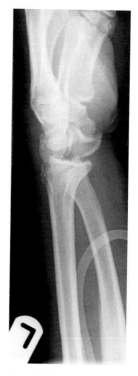

Perilunate dislocation.

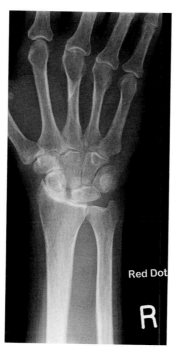

'Terry Thomas' sign.

Clavicular fractures

Characteristics

- The majority are caused by direct force to the shoulder, e.g. a fall. Less commonly the fracture is secondary to transmitted force from falling onto an outstretched hand.
- The commonest site is the junction of middle and outer thirds (80%).
- May be associated with a sterno-clavicular or AC dislocation.

Clinical features

- Patients will complain of pain at the site of fracture and will be reluctant to move their shoulder or arm.
- There may be anterior, inferior and medial displacement of the shoulder in mid-clavicular fractures due to the action of attached muscles.
- A palpable step and fracture crepitus can often be felt.
- Pressure necrosis of the overlying skin is rare but serious.
- Rarely there may be an associated pneumothorax or neurovascular injury.

Radiological features

- A single AP view is usually adequate.
- Often the fracture line is obvious although in children a greenstick fracture can be difficult to see. In children it is often helpful to compare both sides.
- Beware the subtle pneumothorax secondary to a bony fragment.
- In a patient with a history of breast cancer, pathological fractures can occur. This may be secondary to recurrent disease but always ask for a history of radiotherapy as radiation necrosis can mimic a fracture.

Management

- ABCs.
- The principles of management include analgesia and support of the arm. This tends to be best achieved by NSAIDs and a broad arm sling.
- Exclude neurovascular injury.
- Supports should be discarded as pain settles.
- Physiotherapy may be useful in the elderly.

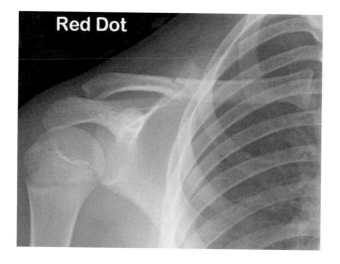

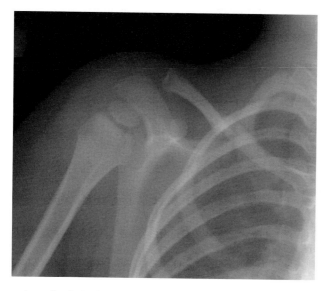

Two examples of subtle fractures of the middle third of the right clavicle.

Colles' fracture

Characteristics

- Originally described in 1814 and is the commonest adult wrist fracture.
- A fall onto the outstretched hand is the commonest cause.
- Mainly seen in middle aged to elderly females with osteoporosis.
- Classically a transverse fracture within 2 cm of the articular surface; with dorsoradial angulation and displacement. The fracture is impacted and often associated with an ulnar styloid fracture.

Clinical features

- The patient will complain of pain at the wrist.
- Classically a 'dinner fork' deformity is seen.
- Marked swelling with associated bruising common.
- Beware associated vascular or median nerve injury.

Radiological features

- AP and lateral views essential.
- The five commonly seen deformities are:
    1. Dorsal angulation with loss of the normal (5–10 degrees) volar tilt of the articular surface of the radius.
    2. Dorsal displacement of the distal fracture fragment.
    3. Impaction at the fracture site.
    4. Radial displacement of the distal fragment.
    5. Radial tilt of the distal fragment.
- The pronator quadratus fat pad tends to be elevated secondary to an effusion.

Colles' fracture

Management

- ABCs.
- Analgesia and immobilise.
- Reduction is generally indicated if there is marked radial angulation or a dorsal tilt of >10 degrees. If in doubt discuss with the orthopaedic team.
- If reduction is indicated it should be performed early within the department. The aim is to restore length, correct the dorsal angulation to neutral or to the normal volar tilt position and maintain in ulnar deviation.
- Closed reduction using local analgesia (haematoma block) tends to work well. This can be supplemented with i.v. analgesia ± sedation depending on local policy.
- Following reduction, maintain position with a Colles' backslab or split plaster and refer to fracture clinic for follow-up.

Related wrist fractures

Smith's fracture

- Fall onto the dorsum of the hand or due to a direct blow.
- Patient presents with a swollen tender wrist with associated deformity.
- Often described as a reverse Colles' fracture.
- AP and lateral views recommended as may appear similar to Colles' fracture if an AP view alone is examined.
- Transverse fracture through the distal radial metaphysis with associated volar angulation and volar shift.
- Look for median nerve symptoms.
- Treated by closed reduction, under sedation, with an above-elbow split-cast or ulnar-volar backslab. Immobilise and referral to the fracture clinic.

Barton's fracture

- The fracture line is *intra-articular* and runs obliquely as compared to the transverse fracture seen in Colles' type.
- Originally described as two types, one with a dorsally displaced fragment and the other with a volar displaced fragment.
- The fracture now associated with the name describes a fragment of the anterior rim of radius with subluxation of both the wrist and distal radio-ulnar joint.
- Tends to occur following high velocity impact injuries.
- AP and lateral views required. Carpal displacement best seen on the lateral views.
- Closed reduction may be attempted but these fractures are inherently unstable and thus referral for open reduction and internal fixation is recommended.

Chauffeur's (Hutchinson) fracture

- This is an intra-articular fracture of the radial styloid.
- Usually secondary to a direct blow to the ulnar aspect of wrist.
- Best seen on the AP view.
- Accurate reduction and fixation key to treatment.

Greenstick fracture

- Incomplete metaphyseal fracture seen as disruption of the cortex on one side with angulation or bowing on the opposite side.
- If angulated >10 degrees, may require reduction and immobilisation depending on the child's age, as remodelling will occur to an extent.
- Refer to fracture clinic.

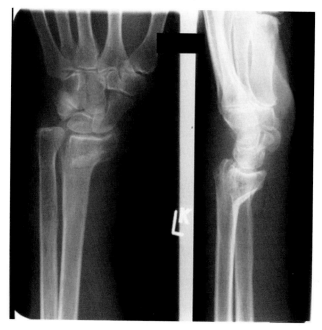

Smith's type fracture.

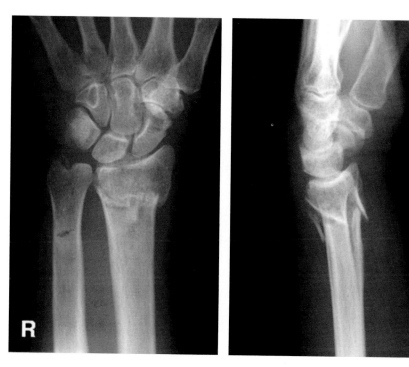

Colles' fracture.

Related wrist fractures (*continued*)

Epiphyseal injuries

- Salter Harris classification.

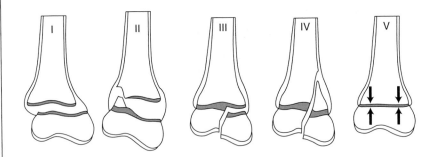

- Commonly type II, with a triangular metaphyseal fragment seen dorsally.
- Refer to the orthopaedic team.
- Operative reduction necessary if closed reduction fails.

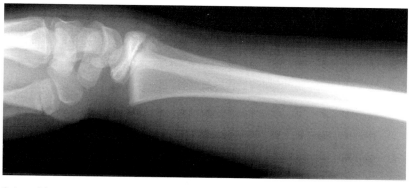

Salter Harris type II epiphyseal injury of the distal radius.

Galeazzi fracture – Dislocation

Characteristics

- Defined as a fracture of the radius with associated dislocation of the distal radio-ulnar joint.
- Again a rare fracture occurring in approximately 1 in 14 forearm fractures.
- Occurs in falls onto the outstretched extended hand in which the forearm is forcibly pronated.
- As with a Monteggia fracture, it may occur secondary to a direct blow.

Clinical features

- The patient will complain of pain and be reluctant to move the forearm or wrist.
- An obvious deformity at the site of the radial fracture may be apparent.
- Tenderness ± fracture crepitus along the distal radius may be present.
- On comparison with the opposite side, the ulnar head will be prominent with associated soft tissue swelling.

Radiological features

- Obtain AP and lateral views of the forearm including the wrist.
- The radius will commonly be fractured at the junction of middle and distal thirds.
- The radius will often appear shortened.
- Carefully assess the distal radio-ulnar joint for widening.
- On the lateral view, the head of the ulna is usually displaced dorsally.
- There will often be dorsal angulation of the radial fracture.
- Ulna styloid fractures are common and act as a marker for distal radio-ulnar joint disruption.
- A useful way of remembering this type of forearm fracture is with the acronym 'GFR' – Galeazzi Fractured Radius.

Management

- ABCs.
- Analgesia and immobilise. Refer to the orthopaedic team as these cases are likely to require open reduction and internal fixation.
- In children, closed reduction under general anaesthesia (GA) is appropriate with careful follow-up.
- With late missed injuries, surgical excision of the ulna head can be of benefit.

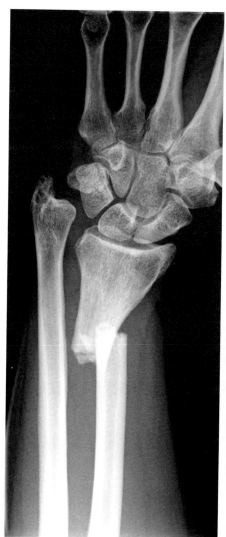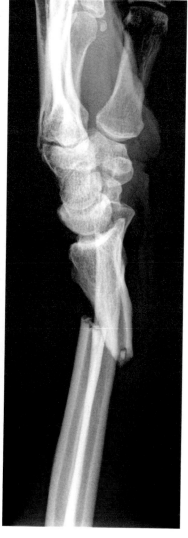

Galeazzi fracture.

Humerus fracture – Articular surface fractures

Included in this group are fractures of the capitellum, trochlea, epicondlyes, olecranon and radial head.

Capitellum fractures

Characteristics

- Fall onto outstretched hand.
- Often associated with radial head fractures.

Clinical features

- May present late.
- Limited flexion and localised tenderness.

Radiological features

- The fracture may be obvious with displacement of the capitellum.
- Subtle undisplaced fractures usually have an associated effusion with elevation of the fat pads.
- Beware of associated radial head fractures.

Management

- ABCs.
- Initial management with posterior splint and elevation. If the fracture is displaced or if a fragment is acting as a loose body, surgery is required.

Trochlea fractures

These fractures are rare.

Epicondylar/epiphyseal fractures

Characteristics

- Usually the medial epicondyle.
- Fractures in children often involve the epiphysis of the medial epicondyle.
- Usually associated with posterior dislocation, repetitive valgus strain or a direct blow.

Clinical features

- Pain on movement and localised tenderness over medial epicondyle.
- Forearm flexor contraction will increase pain. Assess ulnar nerve function.

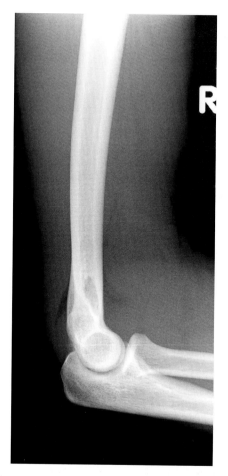

An underlying bony injury must always be carefully sought when a significant joint effusion is identified in the context of trauma. Note the elevated anterior and posterior fat pads.

Humerus Fracture – Articular Surface Fractures

Humerus fracture – Articular surface fractures (*continued*)

Radiological features

- Radiological assessment may be difficult as there is often confusion with the normal epiphyseal pattern. Familiarity with the 'CRITOL' principle (see below) will reduce the risk of error. Compare with the opposite side if suspicious. Typically the epiphyses appear as follows – **C**apitellum: 1 year, **R**adial head: 3 years, medial (**I**nternal) epicondyle: 5 years, **T**rochlea: 7 years, **O**lecranon: 9 years, **L**ateral epicondyle: 11 years (**CRITOL**: 1, 3, 5, 7, 9 and 11 years). Whilst the CRITOL principle does not strictly apply in all patients, the trochlear centre invariably ossifies after the internal epicondyle. Hence if the trochlear centre is present then the centre for the internal epicondyle *must* be present. **Beware missing the avulsed medial epicondyle epiphysis!**
- Careful examination is necessary to identify possible intra-articular loose fragments.

Management

- ABCs.
- Undisplaced fractures should be immobilised with elbow and wrist flexion to reduce action of the forearm flexors. Follow-up in fracture clinic.
- Displaced fractures should be referred to the orthopaedic team for assessment for surgery.

Olecranon fractures

Characteristics

- Usually secondary to a fall on an outstretched hand or due to a direct blow.
- Less commonly caused by triceps contraction with a flexed elbow.

Clinical features

- Localised pain over the olecranon. A palpable separation may be felt.
- Inability to extend the elbow against resistance indicates complete disruption.
- Assess the ulna nerve function as injury can occur.

Radiological features

- AP and lateral. Displacement is best evaluated on the lateral flexed view.
- Again be aware of epiphyseal appearances. A bifid epiphysis is normal although fusion should occur by 14 years. Rounded calcification within the triceps tendon can also be misleading.

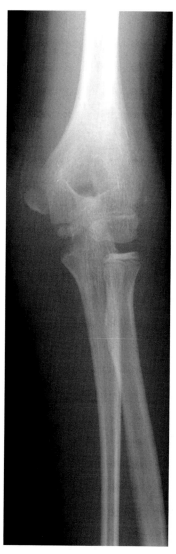

Partial avulsion of the medial epicondyle.

Humerus fracture – Articular surface fractures (*continued*)

Management

- ABCs.
- *Undisplaced*: Immobilise in 30 degrees of flexion. Refer to fracture clinic.
- *Displaced*: Require open reduction and internal fixation. Refer to orthopaedics. Also refer suspected ulnar nerve injuries.

Radial head fractures

Characteristics

- Typically due to a force transmitted along the radius with a fall onto outstretched hand.
- Associated capitellum and collateral ligament injuries are common.

Clinical features

- Painful elbow with localised radial head tenderness. Pronate and supinate whilst pressing over the radial head.
- Elbow extension may be limited.

Radiological features

- Often the fracture line will be extremely difficult to identify.
- Suspect if the history is suggestive and a joint effusion (displaced anterior or visible posterior fat pad) is present.
- An easily seen comminuted or displaced radial head fracture is rare.

Management

- ABCs.
- *Undisplaced*: Compression bandage with collar and cuff. Refer to fracture clinic. If pain severe, a back slab may be more effective.
- *Displaced*: If marginal or segmental, treat conservatively as above. Severe comminution can be treated with radial head replacement.

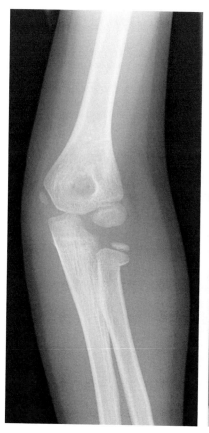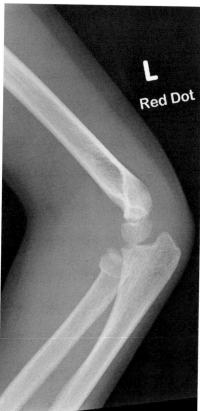

Radial head fracture.

Humerus fracture – Proximal fracture

Characteristics

- Common in the elderly osteoporotic population following a fall onto outstretched hand.
- Depending on the forces applied, dislocation can occur concomitantly.
- Classified by Neer depending on the number and displacement of segments. The four segments described are: *head*, *greater tuberosity*, *lesser tuberosity* and *shaft*. Displacement is defined as separation of >1 cm or >45 degrees of angulation.

Clinical features

- The patient will complain of pain and be reluctant to move the arm. Again the patient may support the elbow with the contra-lateral hand.
- Deformity may be present with associated bruising and/or fracture crepitus.
- Check and document axillary nerve function.

Radiological features

- AP combined with an apical oblique or a trans-lateral view is necessary to identify the fracture, but also to delineate the angulation.
- Fracture line should be assessed according to the Neer classification.
- A lipohaemarthrosis may be visible as a fat/fluid level inferior to the acromion process.
- A significant haemarthrosis may displace the humeral head downwards resulting in a pseudo-subluxation.
- Look for an associated dislocation (anterior or posterior).

Management

- ABCs.
- With minimally displaced fractures, initial treatment consists of good analgesia and immobilisation in a broad arm sling or collar and cuff. Where disimpaction is undesirable a broad arm sling is recommended. A collar and cuff will allow gravitational correction of an angulated deformity.
- The patient should be encouraged to mobilise with passive movements followed by more active exercises once clinical union has occurred.
- Two, three and four part fractures with displacement should be referred to the orthopaedic team as surgical repair may be indicated.
- Fracture dislocations (except simple dislocations with a greater tuberosity fracture) should also be discussed with the orthopaedic team. The principle of relocation followed by fracture treatment applies. Beware as forceful reduction can separate previously undisplaced fractures and thus closed reduction with X-ray screening is advised.

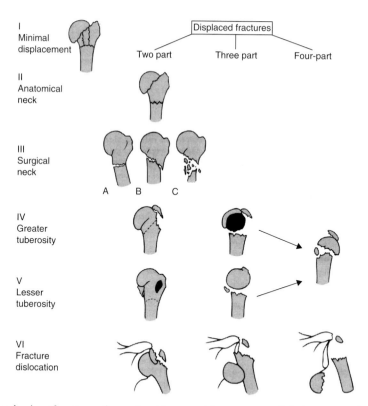

I
Minimal
displacement

Displaced fractures

Two part   Three part   Four-part

II
Anatomical
neck

III
Surgical
neck

A   B   C

IV
Greater
tuberosity

V
Lesser
tuberosity

VI
Fracture
dislocation

Neer's classification of proximal humeral fractures and dislocations. From: *Surgery Facts and Figures*; Greenwich Medical Media, 2000: page 345.

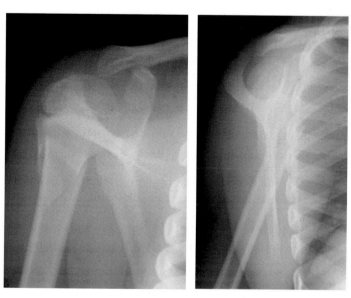

Fracture through the surgical neck of the humerus (AP and Y view).

Humerus fracture – Shaft fracture

Characteristics

- Usually result from a direct blow.
- Occasionally due to a fall, or twisting motion, on an outstretched hand.
- Rarely have been reported after strenuous exercise caused by violent muscle contraction.
- Fracture pattern tends to relate to the muscular attachments.

Clinical features

- The arm is usually supported by the opposite arm.
- The patient will complain of pain. Bruising and angulation are often present.
- The arm may be shortened and rotated depending on the fracture displacement.
- Fracture crepitus is common with complete fractures.
- Suspect radial nerve damage if there is a wrist-drop or sensory impairment in the dorsal aspect of the 1st web space.

Radiological features

- An AP and lateral are essential as a displaced fracture can be underestimated on one view.
- Fractures tend to be mid-shaft and transverse.
- Incomplete fractures can be subtle. Look for cortical break at the site of maximum tenderness.
- If fracture occurs above pectoralis major insertion, the proximal fragment abducts. If between pectoralis major and deltoid insertions, the proximal fragment will adduct. If distal to deltoid insertion, the proximal fragment will abduct.

Management

- ABCs.
- Analgesia and immobilise.
- Closed single fractures are best treated by a plaster U slab.
- A hanging cast is recommended for grossly displaced or comminuted fractures. The cast should be lightweight as a heavy cast will increase the risk of excess distraction and non-union. Reassess neurology post-cast application.
- Follow-up in the fracture clinic.
- If severely displaced/comminuted, multiple, open or associated with neurology, the patient should be referred to the orthopaedic team immediately.

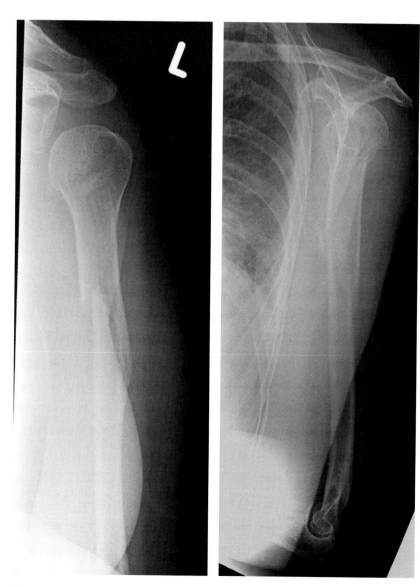

Comminuted fracture of the middle third of the humeral shaft.

Humerus fracture – Supracondylar fracture

Characteristics

- Occur in the distal humerus, proximal to the epicondyles.
- Common in childhood between the ages of 5 and 10 years.
- Usually secondary to a fall on an outstretched hand.
- Classified as an extension or flexion fracture depending on the angulation/displacement of the distal fracture fragment.
- Majority are of the extension type.

Clinical features

- Suspect from the history.
- The child will complain of pain and be reluctant to move the arm.
- Obvious deformity and bruising may be present.
- Unlike a dislocation, the relationship between the olecranon, medial epicondyle and lateral epicondyle will be preserved.
- Beware vascular injury to the brachial artery by the proximal fragment. Always assess the circulation and refer to orthopaedics.

Radiological features

- Obtain an AP and lateral view of the elbow.
- A spectrum of abnormalities can be seen from mild cortical irregularity to complete displacement of the distal humeral fragment with loss of fracture continuity.
- Often only a subtle fracture line will be seen.
- Look for the presence of a posterior fat pad, prominent anterior fat pad or disruption of the anterior humeral line. **The anterior humeral line normally passes through the middle third of the capitellum on a lateral elbow X-ray**.
- Remember to apply the CRITOL principle to avoid missing concurrent epiphyseal injuries (see humeral articular surface: epicondylar/epiphyseal fractures).

Management

- ABCs.
- With non-displaced fractures immobilise in a splint or cast flexed at 90 degrees. Refer to fracture clinic.
- Orthopaedic referral for consideration of reduction is indicated if there are vascular complications or if there is off-ending of the fracture (<50% bony contact).
- Reduction in the department is virtually never indicated and should only ever be carried out as a last resort in limb-threatening ischaemia with senior orthopaedic input.

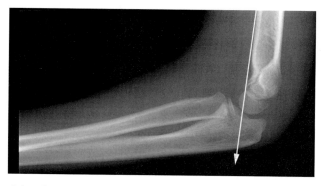

Supracondylar fracture (lateral view). The anterior humeral line passes through the anterior third of the capitellum due to dorsal displacement of the capitellum secondary to the fracture. Note the associated significant joint effusion.

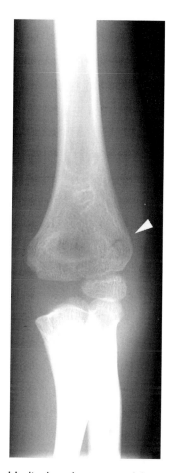

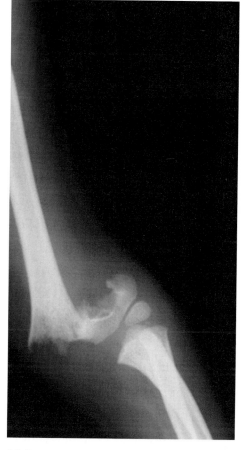

Undisplaced supracondylar fracture.

"Off-ended" supracondylar fracture.

Monteggia fracture dislocation

Characteristics

- Originally described in 1814 by Monteggia.
- Defined as a fracture of the ulna with dislocation of the radial head. Further classified depending on the fracture level and direction of radial head dislocation.
- Rare fracture occurring in approximately 1 in 14 of forearm fractures.
- Commonly after fall onto an outstretched hand with a degree of forced pronation. Can also result from a direct blow.

Clinical features

- There will be tenderness at the fracture site with associated limitation of elbow movements.
- The forearm may appear shortened and deformity from the dislocated radial head may be apparent.

Radiological features

- AP and lateral views of the forearm including the elbow are necessary.
- Always suspect radial head dislocation with an isolated ulna fracture.
- Carefully examine elbow views for normal alignment. **A line drawn along the axis of the radius should pass through the centre of the capitellum on both the lateral and AP views. This is known as the radiocapitellar line.**
- Beware in children as a subtle greenstick fracture may be missed. Always check the radial head position on all views and assess for subtle deformity of the ulna.
- A useful way of remembering this type of forearm fracture is with the acronym '**BUM**' – **B**roken **U**lna **M**onteggia.

Management

- ABCs.
- Analgesia and immobilise, then refer to the orthopaedic team as treatment is surgical.
- In children with greenstick fractures, correction of the angulation by closed reduction under GA is appropriate. Careful follow-up with weekly radiographs is required.

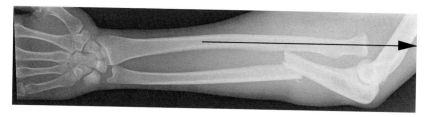

Monteggia fracture. The radiocapitellar line does not pass through the capitellum due to radial head dislocation.

Scapular fracture

Characteristics

- Uncommon injury as the scapula is mobile and covered in muscle.
- Usually due to a fall from height or a high velocity force, i.e. road traffic accident.
- Classified according to site:
  - Involves body or spine of scapula.
  - Acromium or coracoid process fracture.
  - Involves scapular neck or glenoid fossa.
- Due to the nature of the injury, scapular fractures are generally associated with intrathoracic injuries.

Clinical features

- The alert patient will complain of pain and hold the arm adducted.
- Fracture crepitus and tenderness may be evident at the fracture site.
- The injury may mimic a rotator cuff tear.
- Beware missing a scapular fracture in the multiple trauma patient.

Radiological features

- The AP chest film will often show the fracture. Further views including the axillary lateral are useful.
- CT is useful in fractures of the scapular neck and glenoid fossa.
- In 3% of the population an unfused acromial epiphysis (*os acromiale*) is seen and can be mistaken for a fracture of the acromion. Comparison with the unaffected side may be useful as this is bilateral in 60% of patients.

Management

- ABCs.
- Most fractures of the scapular spine, body and neck do very well with conservative treatment. A broad arm sling is combined with analgesia and early mobilisation, once the acute symptoms have settled.
- The same is true in the majority of scapular neck and glenoid injuries. However if damage to the glenoid is severe, with large displaced fragments, then reconstructive surgery should be considered.

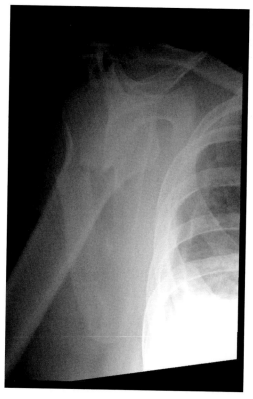

Fracture through the scapular blade.

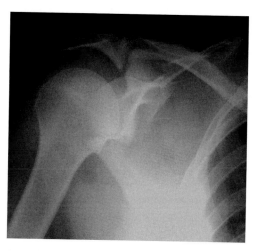

Complex scapular fracture with a 'floating' glenoid and fractured coracoid process.

Shoulder dislocation

Characteristics

- The gleno-humeral joint is the commonest joint in the body to dislocate.
- Related to lack of bony stability.
- Bimodal age distribution – men aged 20–30 and women aged 60–80.
- Anterior, posterior and inferior seen in decreasing order of frequency.
- Anterior dislocations usually secondary to a fall. The labrum detaches allowing the humeral head to dislocate anteriorly.
- With posterior dislocations, the head is displaced directly backwards and is usually secondary to a direct blow or fall onto an internally rotated hand. Can be missed following a difficult obstetric delivery.

Clinical features

- Pain, deformity and reluctance to move the arm. The arm is often stabilised at the elbow by the patient.
- Rarely with anterior dislocations there is damage to the axillary artery. Axillary nerve palsy is the commonest neurological injury and thus assessment of the 'regimental badge' area and deltoid contraction, as pain allows, is essential.

Radiological features

Anterior

- Majority seen well on the standard AP view. An axial or apical view may be obtained if in doubt. The greater tuberosity may be fractured.
- *Hill–Sachs lesion*: A depression of the postero-lateral aspect of humeral head; common with recurrent dislocations, as the humeral head hits the glenoid.
- *Bankart lesion*: Anterior glenoid labrum defect best seen on MRI.
- Bulbous distortion of the scapulo-humeral arch.

Posterior

- Best seen on the axillary view.
- '*Light-bulb*' sign on AP view and widened gleno-humeral space (>6 mm).
- The scapulo-humeral arch may have an abnormally sharp angle.
- *Trough sign*, an associated compression fracture of the antero-medial humeral surface, seen as a sclerotic line parallel to the articular surface.

Management

- ABCs.
- *Anterior*: Reduction under sedation with analgesia. Kocher's, Hippocratic or gravitational methods useful. Failure to reduce under sedation is

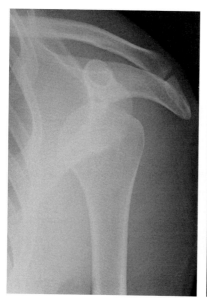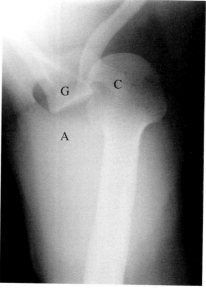

Anterior dislocation of the shoulder. Axial view confirms the anterior position of the humeral head. A: Acomion process, G: Glenoid fossa, C: Coracoid process.

Shoulder dislocation (*continued*)

an indication for GA. Check radiographs and broad arm sling recommended. The elderly benefit from early physiotherapy to reduce stiffness.

- *Posterior*. Reduce with sedation. Abduct arm to 90 degrees, flex elbow and externally rotate arm. Broad arm sling for stable reductions.
- *Inferior*. Apply traction in abduction and swing arm into adduction. Broad arm sling.

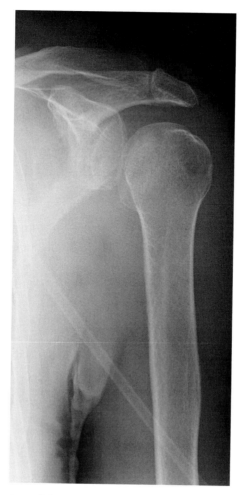

Posterior dislocation of the shoulder. It is difficult to perform an axial view in these patients as they often find it difficult to abduct their arm for the X-ray.

Scaphoid fracture

Characteristics

- Commonest carpal fracture accounting for roughly 60% of all carpal fractures.
- Seen in young adults following a fall onto outstretched hand.
- Classified according to site:
  - Tuberosity and proximal pole
  - Waist
  - Distal pole.
- Fractures through the waist of scaphoid are by far the commonest.
- The blood supply to the scaphoid often enters through the distal pole and travels proximally. Thus in a waist fracture, the blood supply may be compromised resulting in avascular necrosis of the proximal fragment.

Clinical features

- The patient will complain of pain in the wrist or hand with limitation of wrist movement.
- Examine for tenderness in the anatomical snuff box (ASB), over scaphoid tubercle (volar – base of thenar eminence), axial compression of thumb and resisted supination of the wrist.
- Tenderness may be due to a fracture of an adjacent structure, such as base of thumb or radial styloid.

Radiological features

- Scaphoid views are still recommended if suspected.
- The fracture is often difficult to see and an elongated magnified view can be of benefit.
- On the PA view loss of the navicular fat stripe is suggestive of a scaphoid fracture.
- Beware accessory ossicles as these may be mistaken for fractures. An os centrale may be seen adjacent to the distal pole and may be small, large or double.
- 'Bi-partite' scaphoid probably represents an old un-united injury. These are best differentiated from acute fractures by the rounded smooth surfaces of adjacent fragments.

Management

- ABCs.
- If confirmed on radiographs, immobilise in a scaphoid plaster and follow-up in fracture clinic.

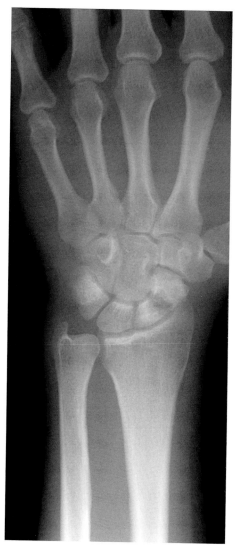

Fracture through the waist of scaphoid.

Scaphoid fracture (continued)

- If clinically suspected but not seen radiologically then immobilisation in a scaphoid cast, with both clinical and radiographic follow-up in 10 days. A futuro splint can be used in such cases instead of a scaphoid plaster.
- If markedly displaced, assess for carpal dislocation. If displacement exceeds 1 mm or angulation >15 degrees, internal fixation is recommended.

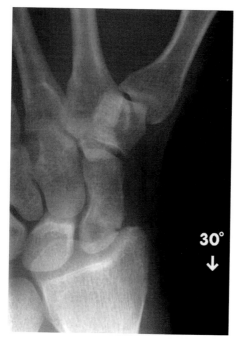

30°
↓

Fracture through the proximal pole of scaphoid.

Thumb metacarpal fractures

Characteristics

- Relatively uncommon.
- Most fractures involve the base of thumb and are classified as intra- or extra-articular fractures.
- The common types of intra-articular fracture have been described by Bennett and Rolando.
- Common, secondary to forced abduction of the thumb.

Clinical features

- Pain, swelling and bruising often evident. The thumb may appear deformed or malaligned.
- The patient will be unwilling to move the thumb and be tender around the base of thumb, typically more distal to the ASB.

Radiological features

- AP and lateral views are useful with an optional oblique view.
- *Bennett's fracture*: A distinctive medial fragment is seen to maintain its alignment with the trapezium. The thumb metacarpal is dislocated dorsally and radially due to the action of abductor pollicis longus.
- *Rolando fracture*: A fracture of the base of thumb extending into the trapezio-metacarpal joint. The fracture line has a V or a T appearance and tends to be comminuted therefore visually more striking.
- *Extra-articular fractures*: They are usually easily seen and are of less importance generally.

Management

- ABCs.
- *Bennett's fracture*: Reduce with traction whilst abducting the thumb and applying pressure to the lateral aspect of the base. Maintain position in a thumb spica and refer to fracture or hand clinic.
- *Rolando fracture*: Reduce and immobilise as above. Prognosis is not as good and requires operative intervention more frequently than with a Bennett's fractures.
- *Extra-articular fractures*: Reduction and immobilisation can usually be achieved relatively easily with follow-up in clinic. Remember the thumb can generally tolerate 20–30 degrees of angulation without functional impairment.

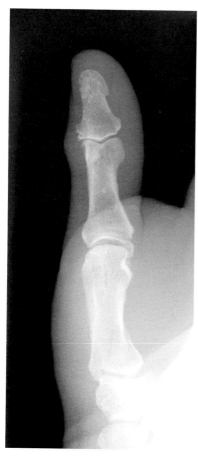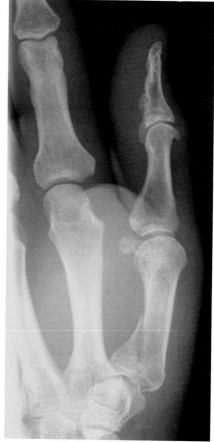

Bennett's fracture.

LOWER LIMB

Accessory ossicles of the foot

Commonly seen and queried on foot and ankle views. Suspect from their position and rounded corticated appearance. The diagram below details the accessory ossicles around the foot.

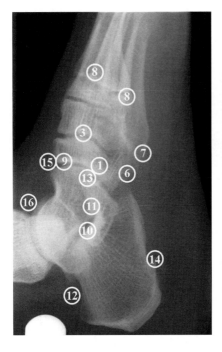
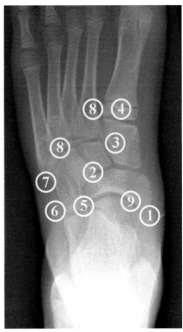

(1) Os tibiale externum
(2) Processus uncinatus
(3) Os intercuneiforme
(4) Pars peronea metatarsalia
(5) Cuboides secundarium
(6) Os peroneum
(7) Os vesalianum
(8) Os intermetatarseum

(9) Os supratalare
(10) Talus accessorius
(11) Os sustentaculum
(12) Os trigonum
(13) Calcaneus secundarius
(14) Os subcalcis
(15) Os supranaviculare
(16) Os talotibiale.

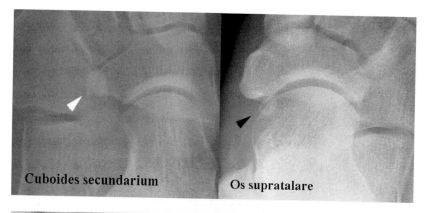

Cuboides secundarium

Os supratalare

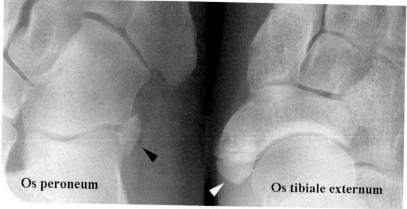

Os peroneum

Os tibiale externum

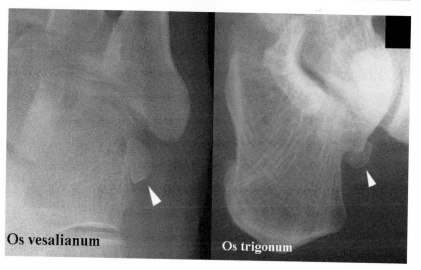

Os vesalianum

Os trigonum

Ankle fractures

Characteristics

- Fractures occur secondary to a deforming force or traction injury.
- Classified by Danis–Weber, based on the level of the fibular fracture.
  - *Weber A*: Fractures distal to the syndesmosis (the distal tibio-fibular joint).
  - *Weber B*: At the level of the syndesmosis (spiral fractures beginning at the level of the plafond and extending proximally).
  - *Weber C*: Above the level of the syndesmosis and a torn interosseous membrane.
  - Note that *types B and C* are invariably unstable.

The above classification is simple but does not take into account injury to other structures, such as the medial malleolus. In addition it is useful to describe which malleoli are involved (lateral, medial and posterior) and to describe if mortice joint disruption/talar shift is present. When the talus does not lie underneath the tibial plafond, the ankle is dislocated.

Clinical features

- The patient will present with pain around the ankle joint and an inability to weight-bear.
- Examination may reveal swelling, obvious deformity, bruising and localised bony tenderness.
- The presence of gross deformity or neurovascular compromise should be treated as an emergency.

Radiological features

- AP and lateral radiographs are essential.
- *Beware*: never send a patient with significant deformity (suspected dislocation) or neurovascular compromise to the X-ray department. Reduce and then image.
- If a fibular fracture is present assess the level, displacement and pattern.
- Consider a proximal fibular fracture in all and image if tender.
- Assess the mortice joint for uniformity. The space between the medial malleolus and the talus should be of similar size to that between the distal tibial surface and the talus.
- Assess the distal tibio-fibular distance as a guide to syndesmosis/inferior tibio-fibular ligament disruption.

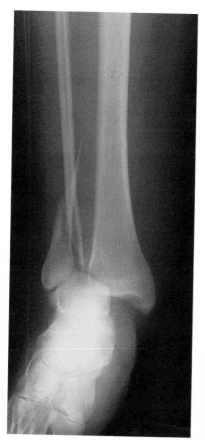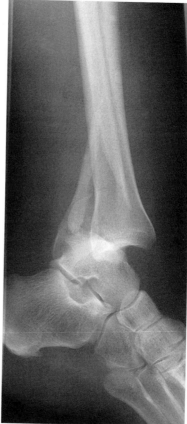

Fracture–dislocation of the right ankle. This is an X-ray you should never see (see text).

Ankle fractures (*continued*)

Management

- ABCs.
- Initial treatment involves early immobilisation, elevation and ice.
- If gross deformity/skin tenting or neurovascular deficit early reduction with sedation required.
- Definitive treatment aims to achieve and hold the perfect reduction.
- In general, all displaced/potentially unstable fractures require orthopaedic consult. These include all bi- or trimalleolar fractures and unimalleolar fractures with contra-lateral ligament damage. Step deformities of the articular suface also warrant referral. Be guided by local practice.

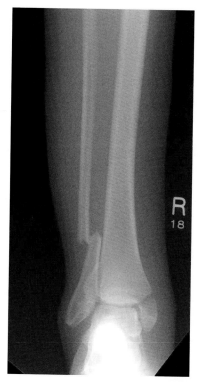

Weber C ankle fracture.

Calcaneal fractures

Characteristics

- Commonest (and largest) of the tarsal bones to fracture.
- Ninety-five per cent occur in adults and are often bilateral.
- Axial loading forces, such as a fall from a height, is the commonest mechanism of injury.
- Due to the mechanism of injury there are often multiple associated injuries, such as a calcaneal fracture on the opposite side, femoral and acetabular fractures as well as compression fractures of the spine.
- Often classified as intra- or extra-articular fractures.

Clinical features

- Suspect from the history, such as a fall from height.
- Pain and swelling are commonly associated with inability to weight-bear.
- The heel may appear shortened and widened when viewed from behind.
- Bruising extending along the sole tends to differentiate from an ankle fracture.
- Beware of compartment syndrome.

Radiological features

- AP and lateral views of the ankle should be performed. The AP view allows visualisation of the calcaneo-cuboid joint and the antero-superior calcaneus. The lateral best visualises the posterior facet and is useful to demonstrate compression.
- Subtle compression fractures can be suspected by assessing Boehler's angle (see diagram). If decreased below 28–40%, a fracture should be suspected. Comparison with the unaffected side (if not fractured!) can be helpful.
- An axial view of the calcaneum, if tolerated, can help visualise the fracture.
- Due to the complex nature of calcaneal fractures, plain radiographs often underestimate the degree of damage. CT is extremely useful both to assess injury but also in planning reconstruction.

Management

- ABCs.
- Early analgesia and elevation.
- Consult the orthopaedic team with intra-articular or displaced calcaneal fractures.
- Controversy exists as to whether surgical or conservative management is best in the majority of cases.
- Good physiotherapy is essential following either form of management.

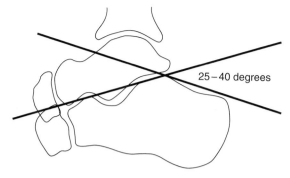

Diagramatic representation of Boehler's angle.

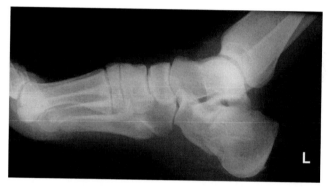

Lateral view of a calcaneal fracture.

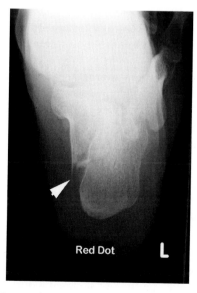

Dedicated calcaneal view. Arrow: fracture.

Dislocation of hip – Traumatic

Characteristics

- Mechanism of injury usually involves massive force transmitted along the femoral shaft, e.g. a dashboard injury in a road traffic accidents or a back injury in someone kneeling.
- Posterior dislocation (commonest by far) tends to occur with the hip flexed and adducted at time of impact. With abduction, anterior dislocation can occur. Central dislocation occurs with medial displacement of the femoral head through or partially through a fragmented acetabulum.
- Often associated with other injuries, such as a patellar fracture or posterior acetabular hip fracture.

Clinical features

- Classically with a posterior dislocation the hip is flexed, shortened, adducted and internally rotated (compare to a femoral neck fracture).
- Pain tends to be excruciating. May spontaneously reduce if associated with an acetabular fracture.
- An associated femoral shaft fracture may mask the classical deformity.
- Sciatic nerve injuries are common (traction and compression).

Radiological features

- Abnormality usually obvious on the AP view. Lateral view recommended in all cases to aid in determining posterior or anterior dislocation and to visualise difficult dislocations.
- With posterior dislocations the femoral head appears smaller than the unaffected side on the AP view and conversely with anterior it appears larger (related to magnification in the same way the heart appears larger on an AP film).
- Look for the lesser trochanter – overlies the femoral shaft in posterior dislocations whereas seen in profile with anterior (relates to internal/external rotation).
- Look for acetabular involvement as this affects likelihood of sciatic nerve damage, stability and long-term functional outcome.
- Always assess the pelvic ring fully as associated fractures/disruption are common.

Management

- ABCs.
- Early reduction is the definitive treatment. Complete muscle relaxation is desirable and thus reduces under a GA with screening.
- If a delay is envisaged, one attempt at closed reduction in the emergency department can be performed with sedation.

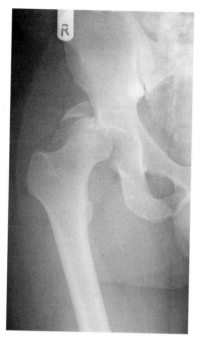

Posterior dislocation of the right hip. Note the acetabular posterior column fracture.

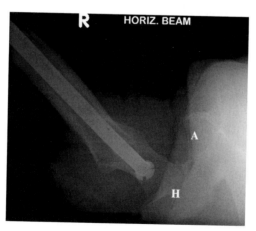

Lateral view demonstrating posterior dislocation. A: acetabulum, H: femoral head.

- A technique for reduction involves flexing the knee to 90 degrees, gently correcting the adduction and internal rotation deformity followed by lifting of the femur forwards (upwards in the supine patient). This is best done standing above the patient with an assistant to stabilise the pelvis.
- Post-reduction – skin traction in abduction, check radiograph and admit.

Femoral neck fracture

Characteristics

- Increasing incidence with age is thought to be secondary to bone density loss.
- Commoner in elderly females; below the age of 60, men are affected more frequently (usually extracapsular fractures).
- Seen more commonly in patients taking a variety of medications, such as corticosteroids, thyroxine, phenytoin and frusemide.
- Most related to only minor trauma.
- Divide neck of femur (NOF) fractures into intra- (blood supply to femoral head damaged) and extra-Capsular (blood supply intact). They are further classified by anatomical level. *Intracapsular* subdivided into subcapital, transcervical and basicervical. *Extracapsular* relates to pertrochanteric (or intertrochanteric) fractures.
- Intracapsular fractures are classified according to Garden – Grades 1–4:
    1. *Incomplete*: Inferior cortex is not completely broken.
    2. *Complete*: Inferior cortex also clearly broken. Trabecular pattern interrupted but not angulated.
    3. *Slightly displaced*: Angulated trabecular pattern.
    4. *Fully displaced*: Severest grade. Often no bony continuity.

Clinical features

- Inability to weight-bear. Beware as occasionally the patient can mobilise.
- Classically the leg is shortened and externally rotated.
- Pain on rotation and tenderness over the femoral neck.

Radiological features

- AP and lateral radiographs will usually visualise the fracture line.
- Look for asymmetry. Compare Shenton's lines on the AP view. On the lateral view check for angulation of the head in respect to the neck.
- Subtle fractures may only be recognised by trabecular pattern disruption.
- If suspicious, but no fracture is seen, a bone scan at 48 hours or delayed repeat film can be of benefit.

Management

- ABCs.
- Initial management involves adequate analgesia. This is best achieved with a combination of i.v. opiates combined with a femoral nerve block.
- Definitive management involves operative fixation or prosthesis insertion. Depends on many factors including patient age, co-morbidity, previous mobility, type and site of fracture, etc.
- Optimisation of the patient prior to surgery and good quality postoperative rehabilitation are essential.

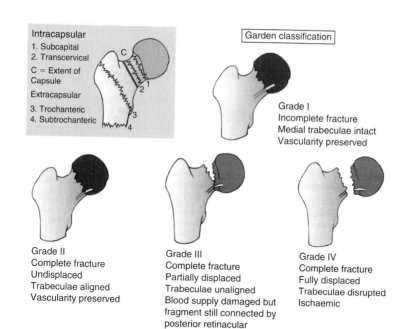

Intracapsular
1. Subcapital
2. Transcervical
C = Extent of Capsule
Extracapsular
3. Trochanteric
4. Subtrochanteric

Garden classification

Grade I
Incomplete fracture
Medial trabeculae intact
Vascularity preserved

Grade II
Complete fracture
Undisplaced
Trabeculae aligned
Vascularity preserved

Grade III
Complete fracture
Partially displaced
Trabeculae unaligned
Blood supply damaged but fragment still connected by posterior retinacular attachment

Grade IV
Complete fracture
Fully displaced
Trabeculae disrupted
Ischaemic

Types and grading of proximal femoral fractures. Note: in Garden Classification grades II and IV, the blood supply is interrupted. From: *Surgery Facts and Figures*; Greenwich Medical Media, 2000: page 353.

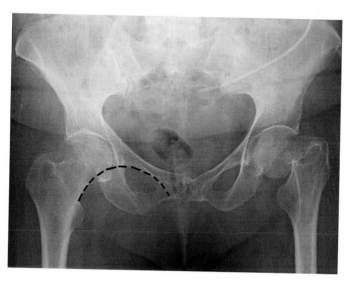

Left fractured NOF. Note the disruption of Shenton's line.

- Early operative management and early mobilisation are associated with a reduction in complications.
- Beware intracapsular fractures in young patients – as early intervention may save their femoral head. This injury requires a large amount of force!

Femoral shaft fracture

Characteristics

- Divided into proximal, middle and distal third fractures.
- A large amount of force is required, e.g. road traffic accident, crushing injury or fall from height.
- Pathological fractures seen in relation to internal fixation, osteoporosis and malignant disease.
- Complications to be wary of include haemorrhagic shock (patient can lose between 1 and 2l depending if open or closed), fat embolism, failure of union and infection.

Clinical features

- Pain, swelling, tenderness, deformity and loss of function will indicate a fracture.
- Deformity will vary depending on the level of the fracture related to muscular attachments and their action.
- A rapidly expanding thigh suggests a large/ongoing haemorrhage.
- Beware of associated injuries, such as ligamentous knee injuries, hip fracture/dislocation and supracondylar fractures, all of which can be difficult to assess.
- Vascular/neurological damage can occur and should be sought.

Radiological features

- Two views to assess displacement.
- Majority seen as simple transverse fractures. Oblique and spiral fractures are less common.

Management

- ABCs.
- Good analgesia.
- Principles of reduce and immobilise apply. Early reduction and immobilisation reduces pain and complications.
- Conservative methods include skin/skeletal traction or the use of a Thomas splint.
- Operative management involves intramedullary nailing or plating. External fixation is generally reserved for highly contaminated open fractures.

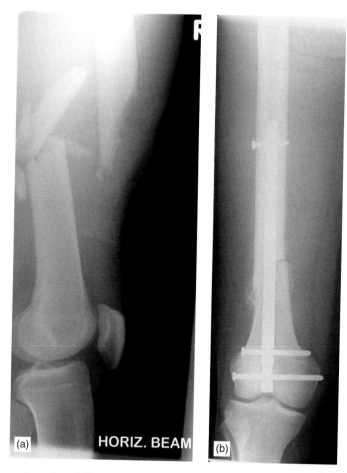

(a) Comminuted mid-femoral shaft fracture, (b) Femoral shaft fracture post-internal fixation.

Fifth metatarsal base fractures

Characteristics

- Commonest fracture of the lower limb.
- Should be considered as two entities as these differ in mechanism, treatment and prognosis.
  - *Tuberosity fractures*: The commonest form. Secondary to an inversion injury in the plantar flexed foot. Originally thought to be an avulsion fracture at the site of insertion of peroneus brevis, although more recently the lateral band of the plantar aponeurosis has been implicated. The types of injury ranges from a small avulsion to fracture of the entire tuberosity.
  - *Jones' fracture*: Diaphyseal fracture occurs approximately 1.5 cm from the base (metaphyseal–diaphyseal junction). More serious than tuberosity fractures. Usually caused by combination of forces produced during running or jumping.

Clinical features

- Pain and tenderness at the site of fracture although occasionally diffuse and vague.
- Be careful not to miss this type of injury in a patient with an ankle sprain.
- Passive inversion is painful.

Radiological features

- Always look at the base of 5th metatarsal in an ankle view.
- The fracture line appears transverse at right angles to the axis of the metatarsal.
- If the fragment is small, the fracture will often involve the joint with the cuboid.
- Fragment separation may be evident.
- A Jones' fracture classically extends into the inter-metatarsal joint.
- Do not confuse with the epiphyseal plate in children. This is aligned parallel to the shaft. With this in mind a fracture through the epiphysis can occur.

Management

- ABCs.
- *Tuberosity fractures*: Treat symptomatically. If pain is slight the patient can usually be discharged with a compression support and advice. If marked pain a walking plaster is advised for 2–3 weeks.
- *Jones' fracture*: Due to risk of non-union and avascular necrosis, orthopaedic referral is recommended. Treatment with a non-weight-bearing cast for 6–8 weeks recommended. Early internal fixation is advised by many due to complication rate.

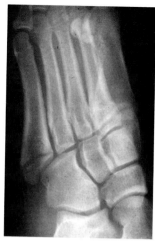

Base of 5th metatarsal fracture.

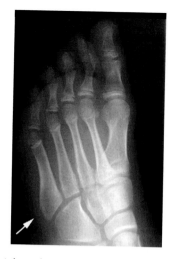

Partial avulsion of the apophysis at the base of 5th metatarsal.

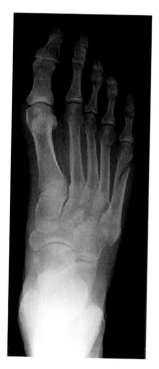

Spiral fracture of the fifth metatarsal.

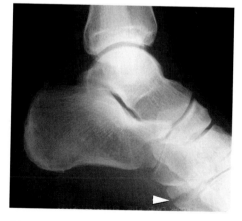

Always remember to examine the base of the 5th metatarsal on an ankle X-ray.

Irritable hip

Characteristics

- A transient synovitis.
- The commonest cause for non-traumatic hip pain.
- Usually unilateral with an unknown cause.
- Age range of 9 months to 18 years with a peak at 5 years.
- Many patients have an antecedent illness, such as a respiratory tract infection.
- **Important to exclude septic arthritis**.
- Consider TB of the hip!

Clinical features

- Presents in a variety of ways including inability to weight-bear or a painful hip/thigh/knee.
- Onset may be sudden or gradual over several days.
- Symptoms tend to settle spontaneously after several days.
- On examination passive movements are usually normal.

Radiological features

- Radiographs of the knee, femur and hip are usually normal.
- Occasionally a hip effusion can be seen on the plain radiograph.
- US is the imaging modality of choice (>95% sensitivity). A difference of >3 mm, between the normal and affected sides is taken as pathological.
- US is poor at differentiating between an effusion, blood and pus.

Management

- If the history and examination are consistent with the diagnosis and investigations including a WCC and erythrocyte sedimentation rate (ESR) are normal, the patient can often be discharged to a responsible adult with instruction to rest and simple analgesia. Medical follow-up is recommended within 72 hours.
- Transient synovitis is a diagnosis of exclusion. When the diagnosis is unclear or the patient cannot weight-bear, referral to the orthopaedic team is advised.
- Admission for traction splintage is seldom required.

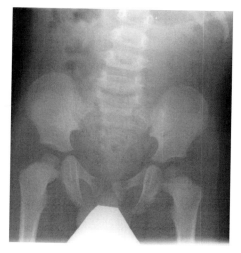

Beware, the plain radiograph may appear normal.

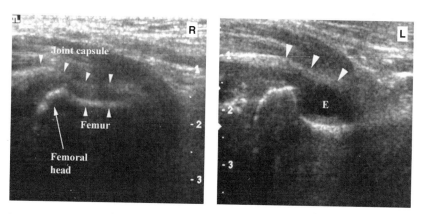

However the US demonstrates a significant a left hip effusion (E).

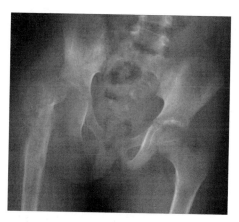

End result of a missed right septic arthritis.

Lisfranc injury

Characteristics

- Lisfranc's joint is made up of the tarso-metatarsal joints and thus a dislocation or fracture–dislocation of this region is termed a Lisfranc injury.
- This joint is intrinsically stable due to the shape of the articulating bones and the strong ligamentous support that surrounds. Thus an injury to this area requires a great deal of force.
- Mechanism of injury tends to involve a rotational force with a fixed forefoot, axial loading or a crush injury.
- Most occur due to road traffic accidents and sporting injuries although surprisingly one-third arise from a seemingly trivial injury.
- The majority of injuries are closed.
- Classified as homolateral or divergent.
  - *Homolateral*: The metatarsals are laterally displaced in the same direction.
  - *Divergent*: Lateral dislocation of metatarsals two to five with medial dislocation of the 1st metatarsal.

Clinical features

- Suspect from the history. Beware a patient who complains of a sprained ankle with forefoot tenderness.
- Severe pain in the forefoot, with an inability to weight-bear, is common. Associated bruising and deformity may be present.
- Paraesthesia may be present, and with severe soft tissue injuries, suspect compartment syndrome.

Radiological features

- Methodical assessment of alignment, soft tissues and bony contours are essential.
- AP, oblique and lateral views are useful. The AP view shows alignment and associated fractures (commonly base of 2nd) whereas the lateral is useful to assess dorsal or plantar shift. The oblique view is useful to check tarso-metatarsal alignment.
- If a fracture is present and alignment appears normal, a spontaneously reduced dislocation may have occurred and stress views should be obtained (often under GA).
- If all radiographs are normal and the history and examination are suggestive, a sprain of the Lisfranc ligamentous complex is likely.

Management

- ABCs.
- Orthopaedic consult as most will require reduction and internal fixation.
- Lisfranc ligamentous sprains require a below knee cast and orthopaedic assessment as an outpatient.

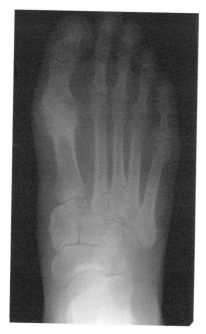

Homolateral Lisfranc's fracture.

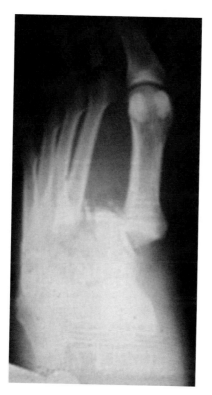

Divergent Lisfranc's fracture.

Patella fracture

Characteristics

- Largest sesamoid bone in the body. Forms part of the extensor mechanism of the knee and is held in place by the patellar tendon, quadriceps tendon and the adjacent retinaculae.
- Classified according to site and appearance – longitudinal, transverse, stellate, marginal, polar or osteochondral fractures.
- All except small rim avulsions are thought of as intracapsular.
- Usually due to direct force, such as the knee striking the dashboard in a road traffic accident or a heavy object falling on the knee.
- May also be caused by an indirect force, such as severe muscular contraction. This can also cause patellar tendon rupture, quadriceps tears or avulsion of the tibial tuberosity.
- The commonest fracture is the transverse type resulting from a powerful muscular contraction transmitted to the patella. This type is commonly displaced.

Clinical features

- Suspect from mechanism of injury.
- Most cases show an inability to extend the knee although this may be preserved.
- Clinical examination may reveal bruising or abrasions, a palpable step at the site of tenderness or proximal displacement of the patella.
- Beware of associated injuries, such as a femoral neck/shaft fracture or femoral head dislocation.

Radiological features

- AP and lateral views are essential. In some cases a skyline view is helpful but often difficult to obtain in the acute stage as knee flexion is required.
- The fracture is usually obvious. Look for associated lipohaemarthrosis on the horizontal beam lateral.
- Beware the congenital bi-partite and multi-partite patella; usually occur at the superolateral aspect of the patella. In these the fragments tend to be rounded and corticated as compared to the sharp non-sclerotic margins in a fracture.
- MRI is useful in subtle cases.

Management

- ABCs.
- *Vertical fractures*: Usually undisplaced and stable. Treat with a cylinder cast for 6 weeks. There is a trend towards splintage and earlier mobilisation.

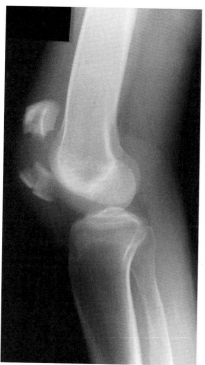 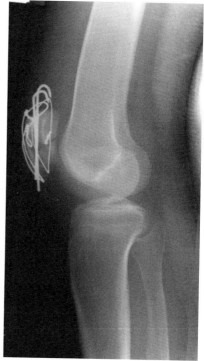

Transverse patella fracture pre- and post-internal fixation.

- *Undisplaced horizontal fractures*: Cylinder cast but follow up to assess for displacement.
- *Displaced horizontal fractures*: Will require exploration to assess the extent of the injury ± internal fixation.

Pelvis fracture

Characteristics

- Usually secondary to massive force, such as a road traffic accident or fall from a height.
- May be associated with vascular, soft tissue and visceral injuries.
- If the pelvic ring is broken in two places the fracture is likely to be unstable – do not forget the sacro-iliac joint as a site of disruption.
- Isolated ring fractures tend to be stable.

Tile classification:

A – *Stable*: Not involving the pelvic ring (e.g. avulsion fractures) or minimally displaced involving the pelvic ring (pubic rami fractures).

B – *Vertically stable, rotationally unstable*: AP compression (open book) and lateral compression (e.g. rami fracture with associated crushing injury of the sacro-iliac joint).

C – *Unstable*: Disruption of the pelvic ring at two or more levels (e.g. bilateral rami fractures or pubic symphysis disruption).

Clinical features

- Suspect from history.
- Haemorrhagic shock is commonly seen due to vascular nature of the pelvic bones, closely related large vessels and large associated muscle groups.
- Shock is often compounded by haemorrhage from associated injuries in the thorax, abdomen and extremities.
- Beware urogenital and rectal disruption – look for perineal bruising, high or impalpable prostate and blood at the urethral meatus.
- Gentle pelvic testing may reveal instability. Avoid repeated examination.
- In the elderly, they may present in a similar fashion to a suspected NOF fracture.

Radiological features

- Obtain pelvic views in multiple trauma and with unexplained shock following trauma.
- Assess the pelvic 'rings' for steps or asymmetry.
- Compare like for like bearing in mind rotational differences.
- Always closely examine the pubic rami and acetabulae in the elderly patient with a suspected NOF fracture.
- CT is a very useful modality to assess severity, reveal associated injuries and assist in the planning of surgery.

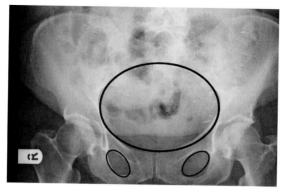

Remember to assess the pelvic 'rings' for steps and asymmetry.

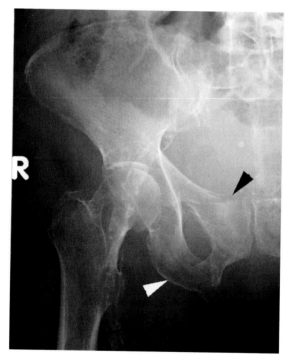

Superior and inferior pubic rami fractures.

Pelvis fracture (continued)

Management

- ABCs.
- Simple pubic rami fractures can often be discharged with analgesia following assessment of their home situation.
- Unstable fractures require adequate fluid resuscitation and early fixation. External fixation within the A&E department can be undertaken by experienced personnel.
- Always consider other potential injuries, such as urethral or rectal disruption.

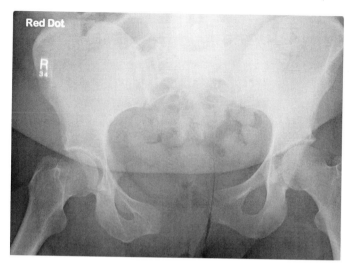

Symphyseal diastasis.

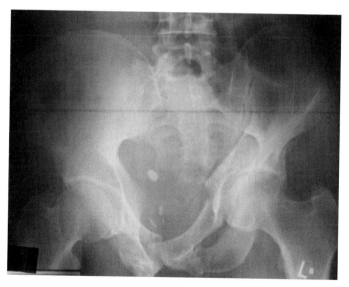

Pelvic fracture following a road traffic accident.

Perthes disease

Characteristics

- A form of aseptic necrosis of the femoral head, probably secondary to disruption of the blood supply to the femoral epiphysis.
- Commonest between the years of 4 and 8.
- Male predominance with a ratio of 5 to 1.
- Occurs in 1 in 10,000 and is bilateral in 10%.

Clinical features

- Presents with a limp or, or if bilateral, with a painful gait.
- Pain may be referred to the knee or medial thigh.
- On examination, hip abduction and internal rotation are limited.
- Onset may be insidious and thus the child may present late with shortening on the affected side and disuse atrophy of muscle.

Radiological features

- Radiographic features are usually well seen by time of presentation.
- Femoral epiphysis appears smaller on the affected side.
- Femoral head sclerosis with adjacent bone demineralisation.
- Slight widening of the joint space.
- Metaphyseal lucent areas.
- Subchondral fracture best seen on the frog view.
- Sclerotic fragmentation of the femoral head.
- Coxa magna – widened flatter femoral head secondary to remodelling.
- CT may show loss of normal trabecular pattern.
- Bone scan will show decreased uptake followed by increased uptake as repair and secondary degenerative change predominate.
- MRI is sensitive, again with varying appearances depending on the stage.

Management

- Refer to the orthopaedic department.
- Initial management involves bed rest and analgesia.
- Later management is directed towards maintaining the femoral head within the acetabulum, usually by a form of abduction splintage. Surgical osteotomy may be appropriate in selected cases.

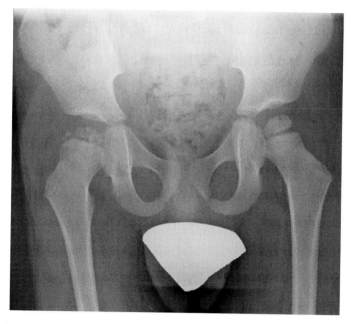

Aseptic necrosis of the right femoral epiphysis.

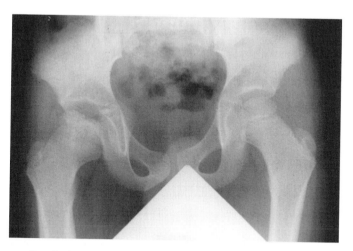

Late stage Perthe's disease. Note the right femoral head remodelling with coxa magna.

Slipped upper femoral epiphysis

Characteristics

- Commonest hip disorder of adolescence (male: 13–16 years, female: 11–14 years).
- Commoner in boys with a ratio of 3 to 1.
- Occurs in approximately 2 in 100,000.
- Appears to be commoner in obese patients.
- Unknown aetiology, although genetic and traumatic theories have been proposed.
- Usually seen during a period of rapid growth when the epiphysis appears to be more susceptible to shear forces.
- A history of trauma is given in up to 50% of cases.
- Sixty per cent will be bilateral and therefore follow-up essential.

Clinical features

- Presents with pain and a limp, not necessarily localised to the hip.
- Depending on the chronicity, limb shortening with a degree of external rotation may be present. Muscle atrophy occurs in delayed presentation.
- Pain and limited internal rotation on examination.
- Considered chronic if symptoms >3 weeks.

Radiological features

- PA and 'frog leg' views are the standard views.
- Widening of the epiphysis with metaphyseal irregularity.
- Postero-medial displacement of the femoral head; this is seen as failure of a line drawn along the femoral neck, to intersect with the femoral head. This is known as the 'Line of Klein'.
- Epiphysis appears smaller due to posterior slippage.
- Slippage may only be seen on the frog leg view.
- New bone formation (buttressing) seen late.
- Late findings include subchondral sclerosis, cyst formation, osteophyte formation and narrowing of the joint space.
- US can be a useful adjunct showing an effusion with early slippage.

Management

- Aimed at preventing further slippage and maintaining function. Always consider the contra-lateral hip.
- Mainstay of treatment involves surgical pinning.
  - Less than 30% slippage – fix without reduction.
  - Greater than 30% slippage – controversial. Either *in situ* pinning or manipulation and pinning (attempted reduction can cause avascular necrosis).

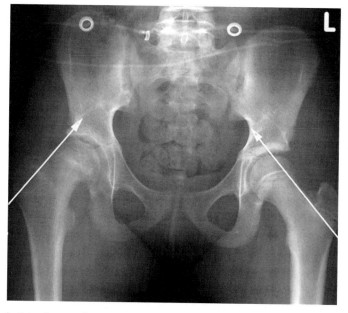

Slipped right femoral capital epiphysis. Note the right line of Klein does not intersect the right femoral capital epiphysis.

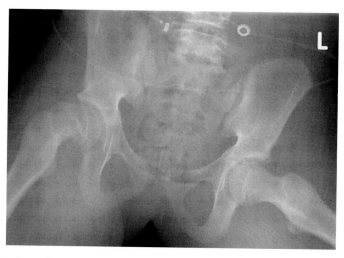

Frog leg lateral: postero-medial slip of the right femoral capital epiphysis.

- Following pinning, epiphyseal closure usually occurs. Corrective subtrochanteric osteotomy can be of functional benefit if considerable deformity present.
- Complications include avascular necrosis, chondrolysis, deformity and degenerative changes.

Tibial plateau fracture

Characteristics

- Increasingly seen in the elderly (approximately 10% of fractures seen in the elderly).
- Intra-articular injury and thus result in loss of joint congruity.
- Wide spectrum seen. Commonest force is a valgus strain with abduction and thus lateral tibial plateau fractures are the commonest by far.
- Beware avulsion fracture of the lateral tibial plateau (Segond fracture) as this is often associated with anterior cruciate injury.
- Medial plateau fractures are uncommon and may be associated with lateral ligament ruptures and common peroneal nerve palsy.
- Classified according to Schatzker.

Clinical features

- Suspect in a non-weight-bearing patient with appropriate history.
- Examination may reveal bruising, joint effusion and deformity of the knee (valgus with lateral plateau fractures).
- The clinical effusion is due to a lipohaemarthrosis and is often tense, limiting the range of movement.
- Always examine and document the neurovascular status as the relatively immobile popliteal vasculature and peroneal nerve can be damaged, especially in bicondylar and medial plateau fractures, respectively.
- Further examination (often under GA and after reconstruction) may reveal instability of the knee if associated ligament damage).

Radiological features

- AP and horizontal lateral are usually enough although a subtle fracture may be revealed on an oblique.
- Look for a lipohaemarthrosis on the horizontal beam lateral suggestive of joint with bone marrow connection.
- Look closely for bony avulsion fragments and widening of the joint space in the unaffected compartment as these are suggestive of associated ligamentous injury.
- CT and MRI are useful in planning surgery.
- A bone scan can help to reveal a subtle fracture if MRI is not available.

Management

- ABCs.
- Definite management is controversial. Non-operative treatment includes immobilisation in plaster followed by hinged cast and rehabilitation. Alternatively, and for the majority of displaced fractures, open reduction and internal fixation possibly with arthroscopic assistance is required.
- The aim is to have a congruent joint surface, a stable fracture, and early mobilisation to prevent stiffness.

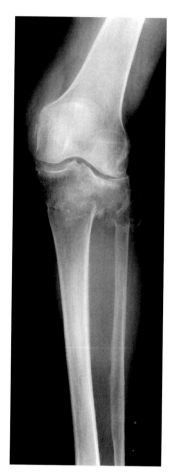
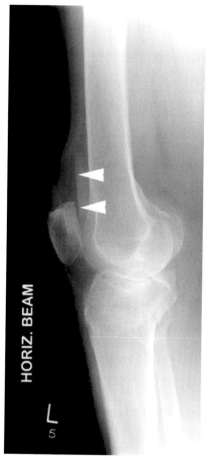

HORIZ. BEAM

L
5

Fracture of the lateral tibial plateau extending into the proximal diametaphysis. Note that the second X-ray has been taken as a horizontal beam lateral. This should be viewed as such (turn the page horizontally) so as to avoid missing the lipohaemarthrosis (arrowheads).

Tibial shaft fractures

Characteristics

- Commonest long bone fracture. *Often associated with a fibular fracture.*
- Usually secondary to direct trauma; often high impact and typically results in a transverse fracture.
- Indirect forces (rotation and compression) tend to result in a spiral or oblique fracture.
- A toddler's fracture occurs in ambulatory children under the age of three. Classically a distal fracture. Mid-shaft fractures should arouse suspicion of, but do not always indicate, NAI.
- Associated vascular injuries are rare. Beware compartment syndrome within the initial 24 hours.

Clinical features

- Pain, swelling and deformity are common. Deformity or angulation may be seen. The foot may be abnormally rotated.
- Although vascular injuries are rare, it is important to assess distal pulses.
- 'Foot drop' occurs with common peroneal nerve damage. Assess sensation in the first dorsal web space of the foot (deep peroneal nerve).
- Ligamentous knee disruption is not uncommon and may be missed.

Radiological features

- Both AP and lateral radiographs should be obtained. Both the knee and ankle should be X-rayed to assess alignment.
- Similarly, inclusion of both joints is mandatory post-reduction.
- Subtle fractures (e.g. stress fractures) may only be identified at a later time from the periosteal reaction.
- MRI can be helpful in subtle cases to make the diagnosis.

Management

- ABCs.
- Initial management of closed fractures involves immobilisation in a long leg posterior splint with the knee flexed approximately 20 degrees. Full cylindrical casts should be avoided in the initial stages due to risk of compartment syndrome.
- Following immobilisation, pain should improve. If pain continues to worsen, other causes, such as vascular or nerve damage, should be sought.
- Open fractures should be photographed and then covered with a sterile dressing. Repeated removal of the dressing should be avoided. Posterior splintage is supplemented by antibiotic cover; an aminoglycoside with a suitable cephalosporin in cases with significant soft tissue injury, additional metronidazole where there is heavy biological contamination. Check the tetanus status of the patient. Immediately refer to the orthopaedic team for operative debridment.

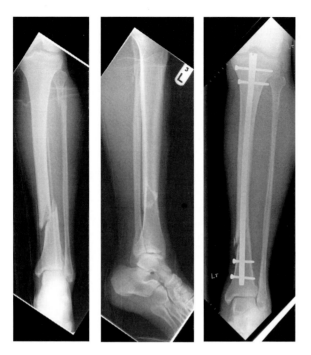

Spiral fracture of the distal third of the left tibia, pre- and post-internal fixation. Note the fibular neck fracture (associated with common peroneal
nerve injury).

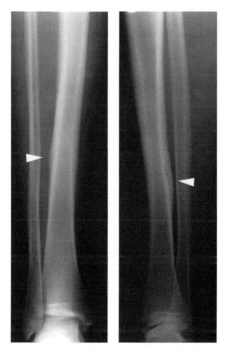

Healing stress fracture (arrowheads).